MW00559354

"The dietitian duo is back! Brenda Davis and Vesanto Melina are my go-to sources for everything dietetic. I am excited they are teaming up once again to address the perennial questions about plant protein and its importance throughout every stage of the life cycle.

MICHAEL GREGER, MD
AUTHOR OF *HOW NOT TO DIE* AND
FOUNDER OF NUTRITIONFACTS.ORG

This book sets the record straight on the dietary issue that is on so many people's minds. It explains what protein is, where to get it, and how to use that knowledge to achieve the best of health. It is eye-opening, authoritative, and practical.

NEAL D. BARNARD, MD, FACC
PRESIDENT, PHYSICIANS COMMITTEE
FOR RESPONSIBLE MEDICINE

Plant Powered Protein offers simple and delicious ways to meet protein needs from plant foods while exploring all the reasons why plant protein is always the best choice. With careful attention to the research, the authors share a message about meeting protein needs that is both science-based and reassuring. This is essential reading for anyone looking to move toward a plant-based diet.

VIRGINIA MESSINA, MPH, RD
AUTHOR OF *VEGAN FOR LIFE* AND
THE DIETITIAN'S GUIDE TO VEGETARIAN DIETS

Plant-Powered Protein is stunningly comprehensive, totally up-to-date, and a terrific gift to our world. If you welcome guidance about protein on a plant-based diet, this is THE resource you need! I can't recommend it highly enough.

JOHN ROBBINS

AUTHOR *DIET FOR A NEW AMERICA* AND
CO-FOUNDER OF THE FOOD REVOLUTION NETWORK

The persistent pursuit of protein is one of the leading problems with nutrition and health today. Questions about plant protein are relentless, as the media tends to perpetuate long disproved myths. Thankfully, Brenda Davis, Vesanto Melina, and Cory Davis have published an extraordinary evidence-based book that puts to rest any concerns. Included are comprehensive recommendations for every stage of life as well as specific tips for athletes. Plus, the recipes look absolutely magnificent! Every person who is curious about nutrition and health—regardless of the type of diet they prefer—should read this book.

JULIEANNA HEVER, MS, RD, CPT

AUTHOR OF *THE CHOOSE YOU NOW DIET* AND
THE COMPLETE IDIOT'S GUIDE TO PLANT-BASED NUTRITION

A scientific home run! This book is the most comprehensive evidence-based answer to the age-old question *Where do I get my protein?* It is a must read for everyone striving to improve the quality of their diet, enhance their well-being, and discover the pathway to vibrant health.

SCOTT STOLL, MD

CO-FOUNDER OF THE PLANTRICIAN PROJECT,
AUTHOR, AND FORMER OLYMPIC BOBSLEDDER

Brenda, Vesanto, and Cory do an excellent job tackling arguably the most common concern surrounding plant-based diets: protein. They explain the science behind plant protein and its ability to support muscle and strength performance in a way that's easy to understand while also providing practical information that readers can implement in their own lives.

DR. MATTHEW NAGRA, ND

PLANT-POWERED PROTEIN

Why Plants Have the Protein You Need

Brenda Davis, RD

Vesanto Melina, MS, RD

Cory Davis, MBA, P.Ag

Healthy Living Publications
Summertown, Tennessee

Library of Congress Cataloging-in-Publication Data available on request.

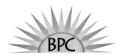

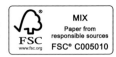

We chose to print this title on sustainably harvested paper stock certified by the Forest Stewardship Council,® an independent auditor of responsible forestry practices. For more information, visit us.fsc.org.

Printed in the United States of America

Healthy Living Publications
an imprint of BPC
PO Box 99
Summertown, TN 38483
888-260-8458
bookpubco.com

ISBN: 978-1-57067-410-5
E-book ISBN: 978-1-57067-817-2

28 27 26 25 24 23   1 2 3 4 5 6 7 8 9

NUTRITIONAL ANALYSES: The nutrient values provided for the recipes in this book are estimates only, calculated from the individual ingredients used in each recipe based on the nutritional data found for those ingredients and using the ESHA Research Food Processor (https://esha.com/products/food-processor/) and https://fdc.nal.usda.gov/. Optional items are not included. Nutrient content may vary based on methods of preparation, origin, freshness of ingredients, product brands, and other factors.

For references by chapter, visit plant-poweredprotein.com/references.

CONTENTS

CHAPTER **1** Plant and Animal Protein: Setting the Stage 1

CHAPTER **2** What Is Protein and Why Does It Matter? 6

CHAPTER **3** Amino Acids: The Building Blocks 19

CHAPTER **4** Which Foods Provide Protein? 31

CHAPTER **5** The Environmental Costs of Protein Choices 40

CHAPTER **6** Protein in Health and Disease 51

CHAPTER **7** Global Protein: A Planet in Peril 62

CHAPTER **8** Protein during Pregnancy and Lactation 69

CHAPTER **9** Infants and Toddlers: (Birth to Age 3) 73

CHAPTER **10** Children and Teens: (Ages 4–18) 79

CHAPTER **11** Protein for Plant-Based Athletes 86

CHAPTER **12** Energetic Elders 95

CHAPTER **13** The Plant-Based Plate, Tips, and Menus 101

CHAPTER **14** The Protein-Powered Kitchen 110

CHAPTER **15** Recipes 123

BREAKFAST AND ON-THE-GO RECIPES   124

SALADS AND DRESSINGS   138

HEARTY SOUPS AND MAINS   152

Acknowledgments   171

About the Authors   173

Index   175

Plant and Animal Protein: Setting the Stage

For plant-based eaters, there are three certainties in life: death, taxes, and the proverbial question "Where do you get your protein?" The obvious answer is "from plants." Yet this answer might seem bizarre to people who are conditioned to believe that the only "real" sources of protein are meat and other animal products. It's no mere coincidence that so many consumers hold this belief. Animal-product industries have worked long and hard to give these foods a protein-based health halo. This book is about removing that halo and putting it in its rightful place—on plants. Plants offer people the most healthful, sustainable, and ethical sources of protein. In this book, we guide you through the considerations that brought us to this conclusion. We show you how to achieve optimal intakes of protein at every age and stage of the life cycle and for every level of fitness. We complete the book in the kitchen, with delicious, protein-rich, plant-based recipes to please every palate.

If you had been alive in the early 1900s, your greatest dietary risks would have been malnutrition and foodborne infectious diseases. Malnutrition was due to food shortages or to limited diets centered on starchy staples. Although macronutrients (protein, fat, and carbohydrate) were discovered by the mid-1800s, it was not until the first half of the twentieth century that vitamins and various minerals were identified. The turn of the twentieth century also brought to light the connection between unsanitary food handling and infectious diseases.

In 1906, the book *The Jungle*, by American novelist and journalist Upton Sinclair, inspired a food-safety revolution. This book not only exposed the atrocious living and working conditions of immigrants in the Chicago meatpacking industry but also painted such a disgusting picture of meat production that consumers were driven into action. Sinclair described sausage meat that included rat dung, poisoned bread, and dead rats. He told of workers falling into rendering tanks and being ground up along with animal bits, all of which was packaged and sold as Durham's Pure Leaf Lard. The public outrage led to the Pure Food and Drug Act and the Federal Meat Inspection Act, both enacted a few months after the book's release. The improvements in sanitation resulted in an impressive drop in foodborne infectious diseases.

Dietary concerns began to shift from infection control to nutritional adequacy. With the discovery of vitamins, the emerging health challenge became the gradual elimination of deficiency diseases. Families were migrating from farms to cities, and access to safe and nutritious foods was more precarious. From the 1950s to the mid-1970s, international agencies focused on protein malnutrition as a worldwide nutritional problem, particularly in young children. Adding protein-rich animal products to meager diets seemed an obvious solution. Yet with time, it became evident that while some nutritional shortages were due to lack of protein, others were due to limited calories or nutrients, such as zinc, iron, or vitamins.

By the middle of the twentieth century, protein *quality* gained the attention of nutrition scientists in every corner of the world. The first protein quality assessment tool, called Biological Value, was based on the amino acid needs of weanling rats. Of course, people are not big rats. These rats can double their weight in three weeks, which is not a goal for humans! The fur on rats increases their needs for the sulfur-containing amino acids methionine and cysteine. Animal products contain plenty of these amino acids. Sulfur is part of the aroma of cheese. Rats thrive on cheese and other animal products. Using Biological Value to rate protein quality for humans meant using an inappropriate set of amino acids as the goal. Consequently, the quality of animal protein for people was overestimated, and the suitability of plant protein was underestimated.

This elevated status of animal products led to economic policies that favored meat and milk. In North America this led to subsidies for meat, dairy products, and animal fodder. Educational programs and dietary guidelines communicated the critical importance of these foods. Early food guides had seven or more food groups, with at least four groups emphasizing vegetables, fruits, and grains. But by 1957, the emphasis had shifted. Animal products took up half the page of single-page food guides—and that was the top half. The health halo around animal products was firmly secured.

Optimal nutrition was tied to the presence of animal products in the diet. Messages to "eat more" dominated nutrition-education campaigns. And eat more we did! Deficiency diseases diminished. The interests of animal agriculture became deeply entrenched in the economy. It appeared that nutrition policies were improving people's health.

Yet the very policies intended to guarantee enough food and prevent nutrient deficiency had introduced serious threats to public health. They came in the form of excesses linked to overweight, obesity, heart disease, cancer, and type 2 diabetes. These conditions are now responsible for approximately 70 percent of deaths worldwide. The health halo around animal products is starting to fade, and global and national dietary guidelines are beginning to shift. Governments are beginning to recognize that legumes, nuts, seeds, vegetables, fruits, and whole grains can ensure nutritional adequacy without such health risks.

THE POLITICS OF PROTEIN

Farm Subsidies: Started for the Poor, Now Funneled to the Wealthy

How would the average meat eater feel about paying thirty dollars a pound for ground beef? Though it might seem like highway robbery, that is what a pound of ground beef could cost in the United States without government subsidies. The meat industry would dwindle without this hefty government support or if consumers had to pay the real costs.

If you were unaware of the extent of government subsidies to animal farmers, this may be a bit of a shock. We could decrease greenhouse gas emissions by shifting subsidies to more sustainable plant foods. This would seem a rather obvious step. Yet when we dive into the facts about subsidies, we discover the power exerted by lobbies from specific groups of farmers.

Around the world, an immense variety of programs subsidize and protect farmers. In the United States, such programs began with the New Deal and the Agricultural Adjustment Act of 1933. In hard times, these set minimum prices, provided compensation for idle land, and paid to destroy livestock if the supply exceeded the demand.

Almost a century later, according to economists, US farm subsidies move taxpayer money to wealthy farm owners and operators. Health experts tell us to avoid certain foods, yet the same foods get massive subsidies. These include corn (for corn syrup and animal fodder), feed grains and soybeans (mostly for animals), various meats, sugar, and high-fat dairy products, such as cheese. A tiny fraction of its roughly $20 billion annual subsidy budget goes to fruits, tree nuts, and vegetables.

Some subsidies are based on production rather than demand. Consequently, mountains of surplus cheese, other dairy products, corn, and livestock raised on subsidized grains are destroyed. Farmers are paid to overproduce.

Meanwhile, health experts advise us to limit or avoid added corn syrup, sugar, and animal products and to eat more whole plant foods. Heavily subsidized foods are linked with obesity, type 2 diabetes, and cardiovascular disease. More than 50 percent of calories in the US diet come from federally subsidized foods. More of this unhealthy food goes to young and less well-educated people and to school lunch programs.

Massive US subsidies have a devastating effect on international trade. Small farmers in Africa and other countries try to sell their unsubsidized products but can't compete with international prices. As a result, millions of people are left impoverished.

The Agriculture Fairness Alliance in the United States and Nation Rising in Canada are working to reform current subsidy patterns. Canadian subsidies began at the end of the nineteenth century to keep immigrant farm families on the prairies and growing grain. Now, corporations with millions in annual revenue and effective lobbying tactics replace many small, family-owned farms. The number of Canadian dairy farms has decreased by 91 percent over the last half century. Since 2003, the United States has lost more than half of its licensed dairy operators. Canadian marketing boards for milk, poultry, eggs, and feed grains eliminate competition and raise prices. Farmers who sell outside of the marketing board can face jail time. Pesticides and slaughterhouses are subsidized.

Cow's milk was not consumed by Indigenous people, nor by most Asians and Africans. For about 70 percent of the world's population, milk's lactose sugar is poorly digested and can make people ill. Early North American food guides, with an essential dairy products group, were geared toward European tastes. With time, these guides are becoming more inclusive and health oriented. For years now, North American nondairy milk sales have climbed, while cow's milk consumption has dropped.

Yet milk industry lobbyists exert immense influence over the government. Overproduction has resulted in farmers dumping billions of gallons of milk. Billions of dollars that are funneled toward dairy farmers are based on overproduction, not demand. In 1984, New Zealand repealed agricultural subsidies. These reforms helped farmers become more innovative and productive. Australia, too, has eliminated most farm supports. Shifting subsidies to vegetables and fruits and taxing unhealthier foods resulted in an improvement of that population's health.

In their document *A Multi-billion-dollar Opportunity: Repurposing Agricultural Support to Transform Food Systems*, the Food and Agriculture Organization of the United Nations (FAO) explains how to shift support to sustainable food systems. It states: "Public support mechanisms for agriculture in many cases hinder the transformation toward healthier, more sustainable, equitable, and efficient food systems, thus actively steering us away from meeting the Sustainable Development Goals and targets of the Paris Agreement."

CHANGING TIMES

We must switch subsidies from poultry, eggs, milk, and meat to vegetables and fruit. With this, we move toward emission targets and limiting climate change.

Are people willing to change their habits? Studies show that concern for animals is less likely to draw some men to a plant-based diet. Men who conform to traditional gender roles and concepts of masculinity eat more beef and chicken, in part because it makes them feel more manly. Health can be a significant motivator for women and for men. A focus on heart health may have appeal.

Plant-based diets can help clear arteries throughout the body. The immediate reward of preventing erectile dysfunction may arouse even more interest!

Environmental reasons may spur even those who believe "real men eat meat" to explore plant alternatives. A focus on being flexitarian and on gradual changes can be helpful.

International meat giants—such as Maple Leaf, Nestlé, Cargill, Smithfield, Perdue Farms, Hormel, and Tyson—see future trends. They are launching veggie burgers and meat alternatives to feed changing appetites. Real men are saying, "Hey, these taste pretty good!" In the lead are Formula One racing champion Lewis Hamilton, ultramarathon runner Scott Jurek, and ultra-endurance athlete Rich Roll.

For more on plant-based athletes, check out chapter 11 and greatveganathletes.com, livekindly.co/vegan-athletes-swear-by-plants, other websites, and documentaries such as *The Game Changers*. References for this chapter are online at https://plant-powered protein.com/references.

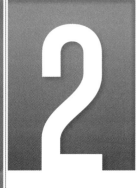

What Is Protein and Why Does It Matter?

The word "protein" for this amazing group of molecules originated in 1838 and was derived from the Greek word *proteios*, meaning "of prime importance." Protein research has revealed answers to questions and mysteries. How do we build muscle or bone? What gives us immunity? How does blood clot?

QUIZ

Are these statements True (T) or False (F)?*

T F 1. Most people have trouble getting enough protein, especially if their diet is plant based.

T F 2. Too little dietary protein can stunt a child's growth.

T F 3. Most enzymes are proteins.

T F 4. Many hormones, including insulin, are proteins.

T F 5. Protein molecules are built of the exact same groups of atoms as carbohydrates and fats.

T F 6. Protein is used for building body tissues but not as a fuel.

T F 7. We require twenty amino acids in our diet.

T F 8. For complete protein, it is necessary to eat beans and rice at the same meal.

T F 9. Animal protein contains essential amino acids that are missing from plant foods.

T F 10. All essential amino acids are produced by plants.

*For answers, see page 18.

MACRONUTRIENTS

P rotein is one of the three groups of molecules that we need in relatively large amounts and that provide calories. These are known as macronutrients (with macro meaning large and nutrients meaning substances we require for life). The three are carbohydrates, fats, and proteins.

- **Carbohydrates** are our primary and preferred fuel, providing energy for muscle movement and hormone function, and for the central nervous system, including the brain. Carbohydrates are composed of carbon, hydrogen, and oxygen. You may have heard "anti-carb" messages, and some of these make sense. Most carbohydrates in the standard American diet are highly processed sugars and starches. In contrast, the carbohydrates from whole plant foods are consistently associated with a reduced risk of chronic disease and increased longevity.

- **Fats** are used by the body to store energy, insulate us from cold, and protect our inner organs. They also are necessary for the absorption and transport of the fat-soluble vitamins A, D, E, and K. Fats consist of carbon, hydrogen, and a somewhat lesser amount of oxygen. They form the membranes, or outer walls, of our cells. The essential fatty acids (omega-3s and omega-6s) are necessary for our cell membranes, hormones, immune system, blood pressure regulation, brain, and central nervous system.

- **Proteins** form the largest and most complex group of molecules. Proteins consist of carbon, hydrogen, and oxygen plus nitrogen. Many include minerals, such as iron in hemoglobin or zinc in the hundreds of proteins that build, break down, communicate, and protect. Several selenium-containing proteins help to protect us from cancer.

Beyond their specialized functions, these macronutrients can fuel our movements and warm our bodies. Carbohydrates and proteins each provide four calories per gram and fats nine calories per gram. We also can get calories from alcohol (seven calories per gram), though alcohol is harmful, even in small amounts.

The source of the macronutrients matters. When macronutrients come from whole plant foods, they are protective; when they come from highly processed foods and animal products, they tend to be associated with adverse health consequences.

Proteins

The range of activities accomplished by various proteins is immense. Proteins are required for the structure, function, and regulation of our tissues and organs. They are present in muscle, bone, tendons, ligaments, skin, hair, and all cells. Our bodies include at least 10,000 different proteins, each doing its job. Here are a few examples:

- Antibodies that protect against foreign invaders, such as viruses and bacteria
- Enzymes that support thousands of chemical reactions in cells
- Messenger proteins that transmit signals and coordinate processes
- Structural proteins that serve as raw materials to build cells
- Transport proteins that carry atoms and molecules within cells and throughout the body

Every protein is composed of amino acids, arranged like beads on one or more long strings or chains. (For more on amino acids, see chapter 3.) The first protein found to have an amino acid sequence was insulin, in 1951. In 1964, chemist Dorothy Hodgkin received a Nobel Prize for discovering insulin's three-dimensional structure. Compared with some proteins, insulin is a simple molecule. Its molecular weight is 5808. Some proteins have a molecular weight of more than a million. The exact sequence of amino acids and the three-dimensional shape are essential to the function of that protein.

Insulin: A Sample Protein

Figure 2.1, below, shows at the left an insulin molecule with its two chains (A and B) flattened and stretched out. Insulin consists of 51 amino acids, and the first three letters of each amino acid are shown. (For full names of the amino acids, see chapter 3.) Sulfur bonds that link the cysteine (Cys) amino acids help to hold the insulin in its folded shape. At the right you can see a three-dimensional model of an insulin molecule. Carbon atoms are shown as green, hydrogen atoms are gray, oxygen atoms are red, and nitrogen atoms are blue.

FIGURE 2.1. The insulin molecule: Amino acid sequence and three-dimensional structure.

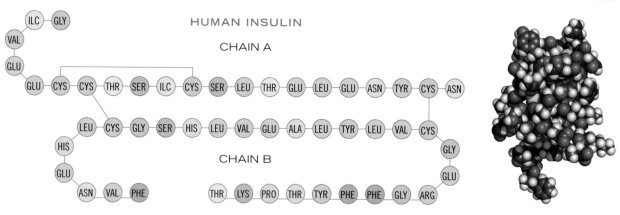

Left image by Cam Doré. Right image adapted from InsulinMonomer.jpg by Isaac Yonemoto, creativecommons.org/licenses/by/2.5/.

Structures for myoglobin, the oxygen-storage molecule in muscle, and hemoglobin, the oxygen-carrying molecule in blood, were revealed in 1958 and 1969, respectively. Protein science is in its youth and new findings are constantly being published.

From Bite to Biceps: The Life Cycle of a Protein

When we bite into well-seasoned grilled tofu or take a mouthful of black bean soup, our chewing action starts to crush the cells in the food. Mashed food passes through the esophagus and reaches the stomach where strong acid starts to uncoil the tangled protein molecules. The stomach's protein-digesting enzyme, pepsin, can break long protein chains into smaller pieces. Gastric acid and pepsin don't attack the cells that line the stomach because the cells secrete a thick layer of protective mucus. The entrance to our stomach features a ring of muscle called the esophageal sphincter. This muscle's job is to prevent the stomach's contents from sloshing back up into the esophagus and injuring its less-protected lining. When people experience acid reflux or heartburn, this sphincter is not doing its job and acidic juices leak back into the esophagus.

For the next hour or two after food enters the stomach, powerful contractions of stomach muscles churn the mix. Proteins take longer than carbohydrates to break down in the stomach, so we may feel full longer with a high-protein meal.

When protein passes from the stomach into the small intestine, most is in pieces called peptides, which are made up of two or more amino acids. Alkaline juice from the pancreas neutralizes the acid mixture. Teams of enzymes from the pancreas and intestinal lining start to dismantle the peptides. These enzymes include trypsin, chymotrypsin, and carboxypeptidase. (We will discuss trypsin inhibitors in uncooked beans on page 14. Can you guess what they do?)

Muscular contractions of the small intestine propel food along. Cells that line the intestinal wall absorb the amino acids from peptide breakdown. Amino acids of the same class compete for specific absorption sites. For example, the branched-chain amino acids leucine, isoleucine, and valine are in the same class. If someone takes a single amino acid as a supplement, it can block absorption of other amino acids that may be needed for protein building. For this and other reasons, there are cautions regarding single amino acid supplements, except for medical purposes. (For more on this topic, see pages 21 and 91.)

Transport proteins carry individual amino acids through the intestinal wall, into the bloodstream, and to the liver. The liver acts as a checkpoint for amino acid distribution. About half or two-thirds of the amino acids stay in the liver. There they are built into protein molecules or are converted to other amino acids or nitrogen-containing compounds. The rest, including most of the branched-chain amino acids, pass into the blood to be used where needed, including in muscle cells.

All body cells continually break down proteins and recycle amino acids. This forms an amino acid "pool" that is not in one place but is in the liver, blood, and cells throughout the body. As a result, we have a readily available supply of about 3.5 ounces (100 g) of free amino acids that have come from food, cells, and liver synthesis.

An Amino Acid Is an Amino Acid

When a protein is broken down into its constituent amino acids, the amino acids become building blocks for various proteins we need for our body. It makes no difference whether the amino acid originated from a plant food or an animal product.

The Miracle of Protein Synthesis

DNA, the genetic material within the nucleus of each cell, holds the pattern for the many protein molecules to be built. Similar to DNA, though shorter, RNA molecules are workers in protein synthesis. DNA and RNA are responsible for the storage and reading of genetic information that underpins all life. Two types of RNA carry the coding sequences for building protein molecules. Messenger RNA leaves the cell nucleus and takes the pattern from DNA to the building site, called a ribosome, in the cell. Then a transfer RNA molecule brings the first amino acid for that protein chain to the building site. Another transfer RNA molecule brings a second amino acid for that protein chain and attaches it to the first. This repeats over and over until the complete protein is built according to the pattern. If a required amino acid is unavailable, construction stops and the incomplete protein chain is dismantled.

Complete and Incomplete Protein Is a Flawed and Misleading Concept

Nine essential amino acids are the building blocks of protein. (For more on these, see pages 19–20.) Once we have these from our diet, we can build the additional amino acids. (For more on these, see chapter 3.) In all plants, every one of the nine essential amino acids is present in proportions that vary from one plant food to another. If we eat a mix of plant foods and meet the recommended dietary allowance (RDA) for protein, we easily get a balance of the amino acids required.

The concept of complete and incomplete protein arose in the 1970s. It was based on matching amino acid profiles of single foods to a theoretical model of human needs. The model is evolving and still much debated. The idea of plant proteins being incomplete is misleading for three reasons:

1. All plant proteins provide every one of the essential and nonessential amino acids in varying proportions. The protein that is truly "incomplete" is gelatin—an animal product—as it is missing one amino acid, tryptophan.

2. The "incomplete protein" concept was based on feeding a single protein source in amounts to just meet estimated protein requirements. We humans are not meant to eat just one type of food. If you tried to live just on white rice, for example, your needs for vitamin A, riboflavin, vitamin C, iron, zinc, and the amino acid lysine would not be met. However, these shortages are remedied by eating a mix of plant foods. In reality, healthy rice-eating populations also eat beans, vegetables, fruits, and other foods. If people ate only seal flesh, their needs for calcium, potassium, vitamin C, and fiber would not be met. Seal-eating populations also eat seaweed, tubers, roots, stems, and berries. On any diet we need a mix of foods.

3. Methods of assessing protein quality and digestibility are evolving. All have significant limitations. Three common systems in use are discussed below.

Here's some good news: We need not carefully combine particular plant foods at each meal as the "incomplete protein" theory of 1971 inferred. Instead, eat a variety of plant foods over the course of a day. The plant-based plate (figure 13.1, page 102) provides an example of how this might look. This pattern can deliver more than enough of all the essential amino acids. Our bodies will pool amino acids from different foods and draw on them to build proteins.

Digestibility and Absorption of Protein

Meeting our protein needs involves two concepts. First, our diet must supply sufficient essential amino acids. Second, we must absorb them. Digestibility refers to bioavailability, or the extent to which those amino acids are absorbed. There are three systems of interest to assess how well this occurs. The first one is the Protein Digestibility Corrected Amino Acid Score, or PDCAAS. The second is the Digestible Indispensable Amino Acid Score, or DIAAS. Each of these systems has inaccuracies or limitations and underestimates the true value of plant proteins. They are based on feeding a single protein source to a group of humans or animals. A third method is True Ileal Digestibility. It involves inserting a tube into the middle of the body of an animal or human to the end of the small intestine to collect products of digestion. Overall, research is at an early stage of being able to measure what is absorbed.

PDCAAS reflected what happened in 1981 studies in which two-year-old children were fed protein. Measurements were made of how much protein and amino acids went in the mouth and how much ended up at the other end in the feces. The difference was initially thought to be how much is absorbed into the body. This system has two significant problems. First, the children studied were malnourished and recovering. Second, the microorganisms in the colon (large intestine) use some protein, so measurement of the final output is inaccurate. Later, adjustments were made based on digestion in rats. But human needs differ from those of weanling rats, which can double their weight in three weeks and grow fur all over their bodies.

DIAAS is based on feeding a specific food to animals, most often to pigs. A tube is inserted into the end of the small intestine to sample the digested food before it enters the colon. The protein and amino acids absorbed by the animal prior to entering the colon can be calculated. Compared with the metabolism of rodents, the metabolism of pigs is somewhat closer to that of humans, though not identical. Also, the form of food can be different. Pigs are generally fed raw whole grains and legumes, whereas humans eat these in cooked form. Cooking breaks down plant cell walls and decreases antinutrients, such as trypsin inhibitors, which hinder absorption, thereby increasing protein digestibility. Feeding these foods to pigs in their raw form doesn't necessarily correspond to their protein quality for humans.

True Ileal Digestibility is similar to DIAAS in that a tube is inserted into the end of the small intestine to sample food before it enters the colon. Understandably, many humans may be reluctant to have these tubes inserted for a study. Studies have been done with pigs, chickens, and rats, though we know the human gastrointestinal tract is not identical to theirs. A limited amount of research has been done in humans that explores the absorption of a few cooked plant proteins, such as soy, pea, and wheat gluten, as well as casein from milk. These studies found that the percentage of absorption of one food protein compared to another varies by just a few percentages. We also know that the proportion absorbed doesn't necessarily translate into what we might see from a whole-food or from a mixed diet.

Is Plant Protein Well Digested?

The amount of fiber in a food affects digestibility. All plant foods contain fiber as structural material, whereas animals get their structure from bones. Fiber is critical to maintaining a healthy gut microbiota. However, as fiber passes through our intestine, it carries with it a small percentage of the protein. If fiber is removed from a food when it is refined—as when soy protein isolate (isolated soy protein) is extracted from soybeans—very little protein is lost in digestion. The protein digestibility of tofu, which has had fiber removed, is similar to that of animal products, which lack fiber.

Although more research is needed, True Ileal Digestibility has boosted scientists' confidence that the digestibility of plant protein is superior to PDCAAS and DIAAS estimates. Whole-food, plant-based diets have many superb features nutritionally. At the same time, their protein digestibility is about 10 percent lower than that of meat-based diets. For this reason, we add 10 percent to recommended protein intakes for adults and higher percentages for children (see chapters 9 and 10). These small additions are reasonable and achievable goals. They may be unnecessary for people eating two or more servings per day of low-fiber, protein-rich plant foods, such as tofu or veggie meats.

How Food Preparation Affects Digestibility

Food preparation techniques can affect the digestibility of the food and destroy potentially problematic compounds. For example, raw legumes contain carbohydrates called oligosaccharides that humans don't have the enzymes to digest. Oligosaccharides pass unchanged to the colon, where normal intestinal bacteria ferment them. The result is intestinal gases (carbon dioxide, hydrogen, and methane), bloating, and discomfort.

When legumes and grains are soaked or sprouted for 12 hours or longer, and the soaking water is discarded, most oligosaccharides are removed. Though not essential, presoaking smaller legumes (lentils, split peas, and mung beans) for at least three hours also improves their digestibility.

How Much Protein Do We Need?

The recommended dietary allowance (RDA) is 0.8 grams of protein per kilogram body weight per day (g/kg/day), which is about 0.36 grams per pound. This is based on a person's healthy weight. It includes a generous safety margin of about 25 percent above average requirements and covers 97.5 percent of the population. Here are RDAs for certain stages of life in g/kg/day: (Note: Adjustments for plant-based diets are addressed on page 14).

Pregnancy and Lactation: 1.1 g/kg/day during pregnancy; 1.3 g/kg/day during lactation (see chapter 8)

Toddlers: 1.05 g/kg/day (see chapter 9)

Children and Adolescents: 0.85–0.95 g/kg/day (see chapter 10)

The following are expert recommendations but not RDAs:

Athletes: 1.2–2.0 g/kg/day (see chapter 11)

Seniors: 1.0–1.3 g/kg/day; for people with sarcopenia (loss of muscle tissue as a natural part of the aging process), 1.2–1.5 g/kg/day (see chapter 12)

Raw legumes contain antinutrients known as trypsin inhibitors, which block the digestive action of the enzyme trypsin. Always cook beans until they are soft enough to mash on the roof of your mouth with your tongue. This will destroy trypsin inhibitors, further remove oligosaccharides, and cause some breakdown of protein molecules, beginning the digestion process. Never eat raw or under-cooked beans. When switching to a diet that is higher in legumes, start with the smaller ones, such as lentils, peas, and mung beans. Begin with small servings. This will give the microorganisms in your intestine a chance to adjust to what will be coming down the tube.

Do Recommendations Differ for People on Plant-Based Diets?

The recommended dietary allowance (RDA) for people following plant-based diets is no different from the requirements for people following other diets. Yet, some experts suggest adding 10 percent to the adult RDA for plant-based eaters. This helps to compensate for possible protein losses from whole plant foods due to their fiber content. This boosts intake from 0.8 g/kg/day to 0.9 g/kg/day (0.41 grams per pound). In this book, we use this slightly higher level of intake for those eating whole-food, high-fiber, plant-based diets. This adds an extra margin of safety and may protect muscle and bone health over the long term. Adding 10 percent may not be necessary if lower fiber, protein-rich plant foods, such as tofu, soy milk, and veggie meats, are regularly eaten. It's also not necessary for people who eat a primarily plant-based diet but also regularly include small amounts of animal products. Larger increases of 15–30 percent are suggested by some experts for toddlers and children. (See chapters 9 and 10 for further details.)

Calculate Your Recommended Protein Intake for a Day

Examples: For an adult whose healthy weight is 135 pounds (61 kg), multiply 61 x either 0.8 or 0.9. The result is 50 or 55 grams of protein.

For a person whose healthy weight is 165 pounds (75 kg), multiply 75 x either 0.8 or 0.9. The result is 60 or 68 grams of protein.

For yourself:
  (a) Divide your healthy weight in pounds _____ lb. by 2.2 lb./kg for weight in kilograms = _____ kg.
  (b) Then multiply _____ kg x 0.8 or by 0.9 = _____ g to get your recommended protein intake.

Protein as a Percent of Calories

When you multiply your protein intake by 4 calories per gram, we find the number of calories that 1 gram of protein can produce. Someone consuming 80 grams of protein (as in Option 2 of the menus on pages 108 and 109) receives 320 calories from protein (80 x 4 = 320). That person may have a caloric intake of 2,500 calories. When we divide 320 by 2,500 calories we find that 12.8 percent of his or her calories come from protein. If we look at what vegans are eating, we find that, on average, between 10 and 14 percent of calories come from protein.

GETTING ENOUGH PROTEIN

The spectrum of views on protein adequacy has two ends and a big middle. At one end is a view that equates protein with animal products and assumes that protein intake must be insufficient without these. At the other end of the spectrum is the view that protein is no issue at all; that everyone gets enough.

What is the truth? Research shows that most adults, including vegans, in Western countries get more than enough protein. All grains, legumes, seeds, nuts, and vegetables are sources of protein, and even fruits contain a little protein. Therefore, it is true that plant-based diets can easily provide the recommended protein intake, and more. Yet in some parts of the world, where foods or variety are extremely limited, protein deficiency is a problem.

A diet can be short of protein if it's centered around fruit (as in some raw vegan diets), is low in calories (as with anorexia or someone who has lost his or her appetite), incorporates too many junk foods (chips, sodas, fats, refined foods, and sweets can all be vegan), or includes minimal amounts of legumes (beans, peas, lentils, soy foods, and peanuts) or seeds and nuts. For the elderly, protein intake can be an issue. (For further information, see chapter 12.) Athletes also need more protein. (See chapter 11 for details.)

Signs of Protein Deficiency

Physical signs of protein deficiency include edema (swelling due to fluid leaving blood vessels and collecting in feet or other parts of the body) and greater risk or severity of infections. Muscle wasting and higher risk of bone fracture occur, especially in seniors. Severe protein deficiency can cause red, flaky, or depigmented skin, brittle nails, thin and fragile hair, and hair loss. Infants and children can fail to thrive and their growth may be stunted. A mild shortage of dietary protein may increase appetite and even cause obesity, whereas severe deficiency can lead to poor appetite. Low serum albumin is a laboratory test that can indicate protein deficiency.

How Much Protein Do People Get?

The National Health and Nutrition Examination Survey found that Americans consume, on average, 88.2 grams of protein per day. This is 14–16 percent of calories. For a man whose healthy body weight is 154 pounds (70 kg), this intake exceeds the recommended dietary allowance by 25–30 percent. For a woman who weighs 127 pounds (58 kg), this is almost double the recommended dietary allowance. In the United States, close to two-thirds of the protein comes from animal-based sources.

Large studies in the United Kingdom, France, and across North America compared intakes of meat eaters, vegans, and people in between who consumed some animal products but not meat. There were significant differences in protein intakes between the diet categories in the UK and France. In contrast, the Adventist Health Study-2 (AHS-2) showed similar protein intakes across all of these health conscious dietary groups. (See table 2.1, page 17.)

Comparing Plant-Based Protein to Animal-Based Protein for Building Strength and Bone

A recent study found no difference in strength in athletes who were getting 1.6 grams of protein per kilogram of body weight (double the RDA), whether the protein came from plants (in the form of soy) or animals (in the form of whey). The Adventist Health Study-2 found no difference in fracture risk and bone strength for men with different dietary choices and none for women, as long as they were getting enough calcium and vitamin D.

What Can Happen If We Get Too Much Protein?

Our liver gets rid of extra protein by splitting off the nitrogen-containing amino group, resulting in ammonia (NH_3). The liver converts ammonia to urea, which is then excreted through the kidneys in urine. Some nitrogen goes to the hair, skin, and nails, where it is bound to protein, forming building blocks. Very high protein intakes (for example, from meat or overuse of protein supplements) can overload certain organs or increase the risk of chronic disease. A summary of 32 research papers linked protein overconsumption with disorders of these organs:

- Liver (excessively high levels of liver enzymes and of albumin protein in the blood)
- Kidney (too much urea, acid load, and risk of kidney stones)
- Colon (increased risk of colon and other cancers with red meat)
- Heart (progression of cardiovascular disease)

We don't find the same excessive protein intakes among adults on varied whole-food, plant-based diets. (For information on the use of protein or amino acid supplements, see pages 21 and 91.)

TABLE 2.1.
Protein intakes in the UK, France, and North America in grams and percent of calories

DIETARY CATEGORY STUDY, COUNTRY OR REGION, NUMBER OF PARTICIPANTS	GRAMS OF PROTEIN PER DAY	PERCENT OF CALORIES FROM PROTEIN
MEAT EATERS		
EPIC-Oxford Study UK, 30,251 participants	90 g	17.2%
Nutrinet-Santé Study France, 93,823 participants	84 g	17.6%
AHS-2 Study United States and Canada, 71,751 participants	74.7 g	14.7%
PEOPLE WITH DIETS THAT FALL BETWEEN MEAT EATER AND VEGAN		
EPIC-Oxford Study UK, 30,251 participants	70 g (lacto-ovo vegetarians) 79 g (fish eaters)	14% (lacto-ovo vegetarians) 15.5% (fish eaters)
Nutrinet-Santé Study France, 93,823 participants	64 g (neither meat eaters nor vegans)	14.2%
AHS-2 Study United States and Canada, 71,751 participants	70.6 g (lacto-ovo vegetarians) 72.7 g (fish eaters)	13.7% (lacto-ovo vegetarians) 14.2% (fish eaters)
VEGANS		
EPIC-Oxford Study UK, 30,251 participants	64 g	13.1%
Nutrinet-Santé Study France, 93,823 participants	60 g	12.8%
AHS-2 Study United States and Canada, 71,751 participants	70.7 g	14.4%

Answers to the quiz on page 6

T (F) 1. Most people have trouble getting enough protein, especially if their diet is plant based.

(T) F 2. Too little dietary protein can stunt a child's growth.

(T) F 3. Most enzymes are proteins.

(T) F 4. Many hormones, including insulin, are proteins.

T (F) 5. Protein molecules are built of the exact same groups of atoms as carbohydrates and fats.

T (F) 6. Protein is used for building body tissues but not as a fuel.

T (F) 7. We require twenty amino acids in our diet.

T (F) 8. For complete protein, it is necessary to eat beans and rice at the same meal.

T (F) 9. Animal protein contains essential amino acids that are missing from plant foods.

(T) F 10. All essential amino acids are produced by plants.

References for this chapter are online at https://plant-poweredprotein.com/references.

3

Amino Acids:
The Building Blocks

The units that make up proteins are called amino acids. Each contains an amino group (-NH2 with its nitrogen atom and two hydrogen atoms), an acid group (-COOH with its carbon atom, two oxygen atoms, and one hydrogen), and a side chain that varies greatly and may contain other elements. The side chain helps to determine the solubility, electrical charge, bonding, and other actions and functions of the amino acid. When built into a protein, each amino acid affects the molecule's qualities. Amino acids can be chemical messengers or help convert one substance into another.

In all, about 20 amino acids are used to make our proteins. These are linked in chains and folded. Think of how many words the 26 letters of the alphabet can make. The very long protein molecules with their 20 amino acids plus three-dimensional folding offer even more diversity.

Nine amino acids are called "essential" for humans because we cannot make them from other compounds and require them in our diet. These nine are histidine, isoleucine, leucine, lysine, methionine, phenylalanine, threonine, tryptophan, and valine. Every plant food contains all of these, and animal products do too, except for gelatin. The richest plant sources of essential amino acids are soy foods, beans, lentils, peanuts, peas, seeds, and nuts. Whole grains and pseudograins (amaranth, buckwheat, quinoa, and wild rice) also are rich in essential amino acids. Most grains are relatively low in lysine while oats provide somewhat more.

- **Histidine** plays an important role in enzyme production, and is a precursor for carnosine and histamine. It is especially important for infant growth.
- **Isoleucine**, **leucine**, and **valine** (the three branched-chain amino acids) are required for building and repairing body protein and inhibiting protein breakdown. They also promote glucose uptake, although some of their breakdown products have been associated with insulin resistance. This is not a concern for athletes, as exercise appears to prevent the accumulation of these breakdown products. This team of three branched-chain amino acids regulates immune function and fuels immune cells. Leucine stimulates muscle

growth and is important to prevent or reverse age-related sarcopenia (muscle wasting). For more on this topic, see page 97.

- **Lysine** is important for growth, tissue repair, and the production of collagen. Though it is present in grains, amounts of this amino acid can be insufficient in grain-based diets when total protein intakes are barely adequate. For example, a shortage of lysine may contribute to the shorter stature of some population groups whose rice-based diets have little variety or have been very limited.

- **Methionine** is a sulfur-containing amino acid. It has roles in building other sulfur amino acids (cysteine and taurine), in detoxifying, and in absorbing zinc and selenium. Methionine is most concentrated in animal products. Overconsumption of methionine is linked to increased cancer risk.

- **Phenylalanine** and **tryptophan** have side chains that include a ring of atoms. Phenylalanine can be used to build tyrosine and, from that, certain hormones and neurotransmitters. Phenylalanine is found in the artificial sweetener aspartame, which is used in many soft drinks. It is combined with aspartic acid and can be found in NutraSweet, Equal, and Canderel. High intakes of such sweeteners have resulted in irritable mood, depression, and problems with spatial orientation. Tryptophan can be converted to vitamin B_3 (niacin) and is used for the neurotransmitter serotonin.

- **Threonine** helps keep connective tissues and muscles throughout the body strong and elastic.

Six other amino acids are "conditionally essential." This means that normally we can build enough to meet our needs. Yet if a person's body is under stress (such as after a burn or surgical procedure), or in the case of a premature infant, it helps to have a supply of these amino acids in the diet. The conditionally essential amino acids include arginine, cysteine, glutamine, glycine, proline, and tyrosine. Plant-based diets, with grains, beans, nuts, seeds, and vegetables, typically provide plenty of all six.

- **Arginine** is active in cell division, wound healing, immune function, and blood pressure regulation.

- **Cysteine** contains sulfur and can cross-link sections of proteins. This makes their three-dimensional shape stable, as in the case of insulin (figure 2.1, page 8). When used as a food additive, it is often of animal origin, though vegan sources are available.

- **Glutamine** has roles in the healthy function of the kidneys and intestinal lining, and in building other amino acids and nitrogen-containing molecules.

- **Glycine** has a very simple structure and is a significant part of collagen protein.

- **Proline** is used in protein building. It gives structural support.
- **Tyrosine** is needed for communications and the building of neurotransmitters and thyroid hormones.

The remaining five amino acids (alanine, asparagine, aspartate, glutamate, and serine) can be synthesized from other amino acids and are also used for building amino acids. Produced in the body, glutamate is the most controversial of the nonessential amino acids. It is present naturally in many foods and in the additive monosodium glutamate (MSG). Abundant in the brain, glutamate plays critical roles in learning and memory. When given experimentally in amounts that greatly exceed normal intakes, glutamate can disturb brain function.

If an amino acid that is needed for building a particular protein is not available in the required amounts, protein synthesis comes to a halt. Any partial chain will be broken down.

Estimating the daily requirement for the indispensable amino acids has proven to be difficult. The numbers have been revised many times over the past two decades without reaching clear consensus among scientists. Also, our needs vary at different stages of life and can increase during stress, such as after surgery or a burn, or when we are adding muscle mass.

The official position of the Academy of Nutrition and Dietetics is that protein from a variety of plant foods eaten during the course of a day can be nutritionally adequate when caloric requirements are met. A mix of plant foods easily provides all essential and nonessential amino acids.

AMINO ACID SUPPLEMENTS

Some experts are opposed to using amino acids as dietary supplements, stating that this can be dangerous. More than three decades ago, over 30 people died and thousands were injured due to consuming supplemental L-tryptophan that had been contaminated during the manufacturing process. Since then, our perspectives regarding single amino acid supplements have relaxed, since the central issue in that case was contamination. At the same time, the preferred source for all amino acids is food rather than supplements, unless the supplements are to be used for pharmacological purposes. Though most amino acid supplements can be considered safe at recommended doses, there are potential risks linked to possible contaminants or to very high intakes.

Amino acids of the same class or type compete for their specific absorption sites. Consequently, if someone were to take a supplement providing a single amino acid, it could block absorption of another amino acid that might be needed. Interestingly, this principle can be used to treat certain health conditions. For example, lysine and arginine compete for absorption. The common herpes simplex virus requires a steady supply of arginine. Lysine competes with arginine for absorption. Supplemental lysine may help prevent herpes simplex outbreaks by suppressing arginine intake.

Amino acid supplement overdoses can cause problems. According to the National Institutes of Health, high intakes of creatine have led to weight gain due to water retention, and some people have experienced symptoms of nausea, diarrhea, muscle cramps, stiffness, and heat intolerance. In general, it is best to focus on protein-rich foods, not supplements, as sources of amino acids.

BRANCHED-CHAIN AMINO ACIDS: SPECIAL AMINO ACIDS TO CONSIDER

Three amino acids—leucine, isoleucine, and valine—have a chain branching off from their structure. In figure 3.1 (see below), this branched carbon chain is shown at the bottom of each amino acid. This trio has become famous in the protein world, as they account for almost 50 percent of the essential amino acids in our muscles. As well as being building blocks, they stimulate protein synthesis and may inhibit protein breakdown during exercise. The effects are especially true for leucine, which is required for the growth and repair of muscle, skin, and bone.

FIGURE 3.1. Structures of leucine, isoleucine, and valine.

KEY: C = carbon   H = hydrogen   O = oxygen   N = nitrogen

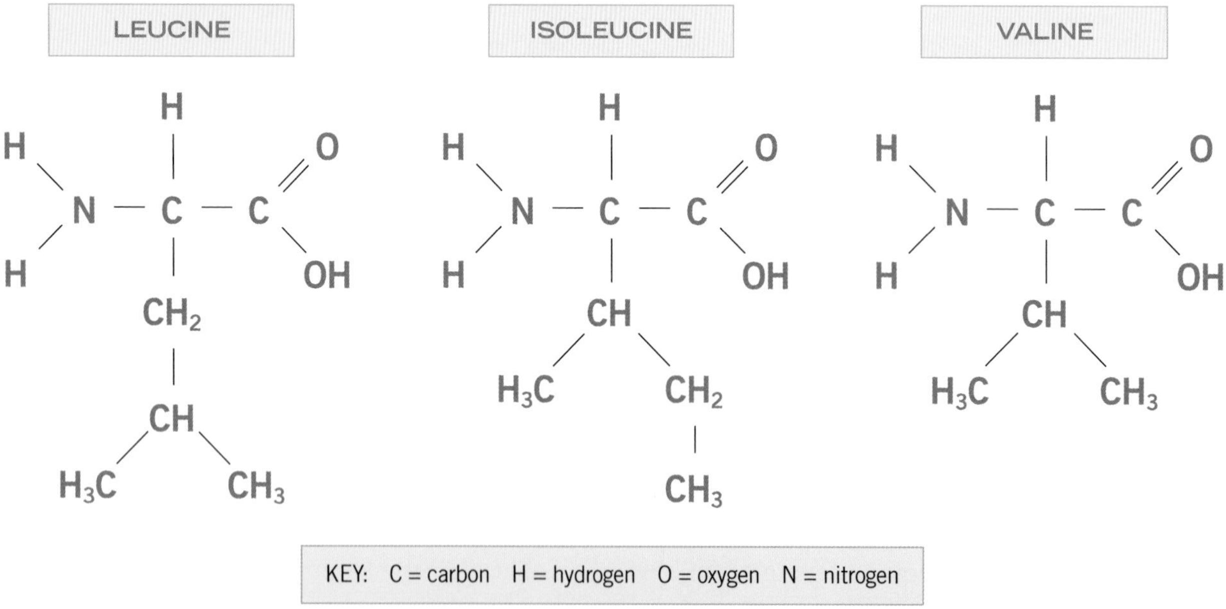

To build muscle or lean body mass, a person could aim for a total of at least 1.4 grams of protein per kilogram of body weight over the course of the day. Many muscle-building regimens recommend that this be consumed as branched-chain amino acid–rich meals or snacks every three to four hours throughout the day. Each meal or snack should deliver at least 20 grams of protein along with 700 milligrams of leucine. (To read more about this topic and learn about simple protein boosts, see chapter 11.) This combination can increase protein synthesis when done along with resistance exercise. Don't expect the same results by just eating protein and watching TV all day!

Below is a sample of protein foods to build in to meals or snacks, along with other foods:

Breakfast: 1 cup soy milk plus 1½ cups cooked rolled oats

Lunch: 1 cup cooked adzuki or white beans, lentils, or edamame

Dinner: ½ cup tofu, soybeans, or tempeh

Snack: 1 nut butter sandwich (3 tablespoons peanut butter or almond butter with 2 slices whole wheat bread)

Other high-protein, high-leucine options are falafel, rice with beans, commercial veggie burgers, hemp seeds, peanuts, pumpkin seeds, quinoa with peas, and whole wheat spaghetti with veggie meatballs. (For more ideas, see chapters 11, 12, and 13.) High-leucine plant foods include legumes, seeds, nuts, and certain grains. Try our granola (page 127).

Table 3.1 (page 24) shows amounts of leucine in various foods. (The recipes in chapter 15 also provide leucine content.) Another column shows lysine values, as these are of interest for menus that are centered on grains such as rice, with little else.

There are smaller amounts of leucine, lysine, and other essential amino acids in kale, spinach, collard greens, asparagus, corn, broccoli, potatoes, hazelnuts, pine nuts, avocados, and many other plant foods. All of these essential amino acids are required for plant growth and function. A plant-based meal will include even more amino acids beyond those foods that are particularly high in protein.

The recommended dietary allowance for leucine is 19 milligrams per pound of body weight, or 42 milligrams per kilogram. As you will see from the nutritional analysis provided with each recipe in this book, the recipes are designed to provide plenty of protein and leucine.

Some athletes may choose to further increase their protein intakes. Protein supplements can be a practical and effective way to do this. Supplements based on hemp, peas, pumpkin seeds, soy, or a mix of these, can help reach higher protein targets and supply a good balance of amino acids. The National Institutes of Health has not indicated any safety concerns for daily intakes of up to 2 grams of protein per kilogram of body weight.

TABLE 3.1. Foods that provide significant amounts of protein, leucine, and lysine

FOOD GROUP	VOLUME MEASURE	WEIGHT GRAMS	PROTEIN GRAMS	LEUCINE MILLIGRAMS	LYSINE MILLIGRAMS
LEGUMES (COOKED)					
Edamame	1 cup (250 ml)	172	31	2,331	1,906
Kidney beans	1 cup (250 ml)	177	15	1,227	1,053
Lentils	1 cup (250 ml)	198	18	1,295	1,247
Lima beans	1 cup (250 ml)	188	15	1,265	983
Navy beans	1 cup (250 ml)	182	15	1,274	946
Peanuts, roasted	½ cup (125 ml)	73	18	1,120	620
Pinto beans	1 cup (250 ml)	171	15	1,308	1,077
Soy protein powder*	1 scoop (2½ T./37.5 ml)	30 g (1 oz.)	25	1,926	1,513
Split peas	1 cup (250 ml)	196	16	1,172	1,180
Tofu, firm	½ cup (125 ml)	126	22	1,754	1,113
SEEDS					
Chia seeds	¼ cup (60 ml)	48	8	658	466
Flaxseeds	¼ cup (60 ml)	42	8	519	362
Hemp seeds	¼ cup (60 ml)	40	13	865	511
Pumpkin seeds	¼ cup (60 ml)	30	9	705	360
Sesame tahini	3 tablespoons (45 ml)	45	8	585	246
Sunflower seeds	¼ cup (60 ml)	32	6	451	255
NUTS, WHOLE					
Almonds	¼ cup (60 ml)	36	8	527	203
Brazil nuts	¼ cup (60 ml)	30	4	592	284
Cashews	¼ cup (60 ml)	34	5	440	280
Hazelnuts	¼ cup (60 ml)	34	4	359	142
Pecans	¼ cup (60 ml)	26	2	148	71
Pistachio nuts	¼ cup (60 ml)	31	6	493	350
Walnuts, black	¼ cup (60 ml)	31	6	421	178
Walnuts, English	¼ cup (60 ml)	25	4	293	106

FOOD GROUP	VOLUME MEASURE	WEIGHT GRAMS	PROTEIN GRAMS	LEUCINE MILLIGRAMS	LYSINE MILLIGRAMS
GRAINS, COOKED					
Amaranth	1 cup (250 ml)	246	9	678	577
Buckwheat	1 cup (250 ml)	168	6	356	289
Corn	1 cup (250 ml)	149	5	533	210
Kamut berries	1 cup (250 ml)	172	10	743	277
Oats (oatmeal)	1 cup (250 ml)	234	6	505	316
Quinoa	1 cup (250 ml)	185	8	483	442
Rice, brown	1 cup (250 ml)	202	6	432	200
Rice, white	1 cup (250 ml)	158	4	351	153
Seitan	3.5 ounces (100 g)	84	15	1,718	430
Spelt berries	1 cup (250 ml)	194	11	621	237
Whole wheat bread	2 slices	64	8	200	82
Whole wheat pasta	1 cup (250 ml)	117	7	479	156

Sources: ESHA Research (https://esha.com/products/food-processor/); https://www.myfooddata.com/; https://nutritiondata.self.com/; and https://fdc.nal.usda.gov/. *Check package labels for brand-specific amounts.

Can Branched-Chain Amino Acids or Leucine Supplements Build Muscle?

The scientific literature emphasizes that taking branched-chain amino acid supplements alone does not enhance muscle protein synthesis more than consuming these in foods, along with the other essential amino acids. Many articles that promote relatively high amounts of amino acid supplements (branched-chain amino acids or leucine) or whey are written by authors who are funded by companies supplying these products.

The International Society of Sports Nutrition does not recommend the use of branched-chain amino acids to maximize protein synthesis, given the limited evidence and inconsistent results. From a whole-food, plant-based diet with plenty of legumes, seeds, nuts, and whole grains, you will be getting plenty of branched-chain amino acids and the other amino acids, plus other nutrients needed for superb health. It is important to center your diet on high protein soy foods, other legumes, seeds, and the types of recipes that you find in this book.

Are Oral Supplements of Branched-Chain Amino Acids Safe?

The National Institutes of Health suggests that oral branched-chain amino acid supplements of up to 20 grams per day, taken in divided doses, appear safe for up to six weeks. Note that if you're taking branched-chain amino acids for muscle building, other amino acids must be available too. For leucine alone, an upper safe limit of 500 milligrams per kilogram of body weight per day is recommended for men (including young and elderly men). While branched-chain amino acids and leucine supplements appear safe, research is lacking on women and on long-term use. The use of branched-chain amino acid and leucine supplements is not advised for pregnant or breastfeeding women. Side effects may include nausea, pain, and headaches. Branched-chain amino acids may interfere with blood glucose levels during and after surgery. High intakes can be hazardous to people with kidney or liver disease, chronic alcoholism, or branched-chain ketoaciduria.

PLANT PROTEIN IS AS GOOD AS ANIMAL PROTEIN FOR MUSCLE BUILDING

When leucine content is matched, plant protein is equivalent to animal protein for muscle synthesis. Nine studies compared athletes with goals of gaining muscle mass and strength in response to doing resistance exercise—bench presses for upper body and squats for lower body. A meta-analysis found that supplementation with whey or soy protein during resistance exercise resulted in similar increases in lean body mass and strength. The take-home message is that if you're trying to build muscle, a well-planned, plant-based diet has you covered.

SOY SENSE AND NONSENSE

No plant food is more mired in controversy than soy. The roots lie in good and bad science, and in the fact that soy foods are a threat to the animal-products industry. As many people shift toward plant foods, interest in soy increases due to its top-quality protein and protective action against cardiovascular disease and hormone-related cancers, such as prostate and breast cancer.

Reliable Soy Science

A major group of active components in soy are the isoflavones. These can have the following effects:

1. For people with hypothyroidism or iodine deficiency, soy isoflavones can affect the thyroid gland. Their soy intake should be limited until the problem is corrected. Solutions involve adjusting the dosage of thyroid hormone for people with hypothyroidism. Iodine deficiency can be remedied by a supplement, a little iodized salt, or sea vegetables.

2. Isoflavones are similar in structure to human estrogen, though they are not identical. More than a decade ago, theories arose that isoflavones might mimic estrogen's potentially cancer-causing effects. Since then, this has been proven false. Evidence suggests that soy intake during childhood and adolescence is actually protective against breast cancer in later life. Moderate soy consumption (such as two to four servings per day) may protect against various cancers, possibly because the isoflavones block estrogen. Soy is linked with a lower risk of gastrointestinal cancers. Soy may also reduce hot flashes and wrinkles. Men who regularly consume soy foods have a 29 percent reduced risk of prostate cancer. Exchanging animal protein for 30 grams per day of soy protein can lower LDL cholesterol.

Misapplied Science

Big bad rumors about soy arose from a grain of truth. Two men who regularly consumed 12 or more servings of soy daily for a year eventually developed health problems: enlarged breast tissue and loss of libido. One man drank three quarts of soy milk a day. The other had 20 servings of soy foods a day. In both cases, without these excesses of soy, their health and libido reverted to normal. But their cases were magnified and sensationalized, creating fears of feminization among men. Focusing our entire diet on *any* item will undermine health. Such imbalance leads to nutrient shortages. Other anti-soy propaganda was based on rats, mice, or parrots eating diets of raw soy, which was entirely unsuited to their physiology. A healthy intake of two to four servings of soy per day is suitable for adults, as is one or two servings a day for children.

Is Soy Safe?

Soy has a long history of use throughout Asia and among vegetarians worldwide. Two of the healthiest, long-lived populations—the Okinawan Japanese and the Seventh-day Adventists in Loma Linda, California—are frequent soy consumers. If soy were dangerous, its effects would be reflected in their health and longevity. In Asia, tofu and soy milk have been enjoyed for centuries. Tempeh's fermentation process further supports mineral absorption. Edamame—young, whole soybeans—can be eaten from the shell after steaming. For people who want to impress their meat-loving friends and family, amazing meat-like products are made with soy protein, which is highly rated in protein quality. We recommend selecting less highly processed, organic products most of the time.

Making Sense of Plant-Based Meat Alternatives

Why would some vegetarians want to eat something that looks and tastes like meat? A wise man made the point that we urban dwellers do not go up to a turkey or pig and take a bite from its breast or backside. Instead, the animals are slaughtered and their flesh is made into human-friendly forms, ready for the refrigerator or freezer case. Plant foods can easily be made into similar forms that appeal to humans.

Plant-based meat alternatives are meatless meats. They are products that have the flavor, texture, and appearance of traditional meat products such as burgers, sausages, meatballs, chicken nuggets, beef or chicken strips, processed meat slices, and bacon. Yet they contain no animal flesh whatsoever. Plant-based meat alternatives are produced using plant matter. Some meat alternatives are made with isolated plant proteins such as soy or peas. Others are made with gluten, beans, tofu, vegetables, nuts, seeds, and grains.

While meat alternatives have been available for many years, their rise in popularity is recent. The plant-based meat alternative market has been growing at almost double the rate of the animal-based meat market. And the biggest surprise is that much of this growth is because omnivores are purchasing these products. This rise in sales coincides with what is called the "next generation" plant-based meat products that look and taste so much like meat, that it can be hard to tell them apart. So, what is the attraction of plant-based meat alternatives? Perhaps the most compelling reason, especially for young people, is that they produce an estimated 89 percent fewer greenhouse gas emissions than meat, thus helping to mitigate climate change. Plant-based meat alternatives clearly help to reduce animal suffering as well as the risk of some chronic diseases. Vegetarians rarely give up meat because they don't like the taste or texture. They give it up because of ecological, health, and ethical concerns. Plant-based meat alternatives allow vegetarians and other plant-based eaters to enjoy familiar foods that have been on their menus for many years. In this way, they can continue to prepare many traditional family favorites.

Are Plant-Based Meat Alternatives Healthy Choices?

Plant-based meat alternatives include a wide variety of products, some of which are more healthful than others. Those prepared with whole foods such as lentils, beans, quinoa, or other whole grains, vegetables, nuts, and seeds are the most healthful options. Those made with protein isolates or concentrates are more processed, but the protein they contain is generally of high quality and is highly digestible. All these products can make meeting protein needs easier, especially for seniors and athletes. While it is important to include a wide variety of whole plant foods in the diet, allowing for some meat alternatives as part of the mix is a reasonable choice. Do read labels to compare sodium and fat content. Meat alternatives are more healthful choices than the meat they replace. Although there is limited research, a 2020 clinical trial reported better cardiovascular disease markers when people ate meat alternatives compared to meat. What makes these products a better choice for health? Let's consider some of the advantages of meat alternatives compared to meat.

Meat Alternatives versus Meat

- Meat alternatives made of beans and other plant foods contain fiber whereas meat has none.
- Meat alternatives *may* provide fewer calories and less fat—check labels for amounts specific to brands.
- A study of 37 plant-based meat alternatives showed that they had more fiber, folate, B_{12}, and manganese than animal meats.
- Compared with beef, Beyond Burger patties, Impossible Beef burgers, and similar products deliver the same amount of protein along with more iron, calcium, and fiber.
- The protein content of many meat alternatives is similar to the animal products they replace—check labels.
- Meat alternatives do not generate TMAO (trimethylamine-N-oxide), linked to heart disease, and don't provide cholesterol.
- Meat alternatives do not provide Neu5Gc (linked with cancer).
- Meat alternatives offer less chance of foodborne illness since they avoid the fecal contamination risk in animal products.
- Compared to a standard beef patty, making a plant-based patty takes one-tenth or less the amount of water and land, with less than one-tenth of the greenhouse gas emissions.

Downsides to Plant-Based Meat Alternatives

Yes, some meat alternatives have higher levels of sugar and salt. While most are lower in total and saturated fat, some contain significant amounts. Many meat alternatives are highly processed, so do not contain as much fiber, phytochemicals, antioxidants, and other protective components as whole plant foods. Meat alternatives can get tough when overcooked. Be sure to read labels to compare ingredients, protein, sodium, and fat content.

The Bottom Line

Meat alternatives can provide variety and can help when introducing dubious friends and relations to plant-based eating. Beyond burgers, Impossible burgers, and similar products are impressive imposters that offer meat-like tastes and textures. Highly processed meat alternatives can be a small part of a wholesome diet. The most healthful meat alternatives are those made with whole plant foods as ingredients, such as beans, whole grains, mushrooms, and other vegetables. These can be used more liberally.

For people who enjoy eating actual meat, there is an alternative: cultured, or lab-grown, meat. While this is nutritionally on par with meat from farmed animals, it is produced without the pain, suffering, and death associated with conventional animal farming. It also is without the massive environmental footprint. The primary challenge facing cell-based agriculture companies is how to make their products affordable to consumers. While cultured options are still more expensive than conventional meats, their prices are expected to decline as production increases. If you would rather not give up meat but would prefer a kinder, more sustainable option, keep your finger on the pulse of meat grown from cells.

References for this chapter are online at https://plant-poweredprotein.com/references.

4

Which Foods
Provide Protein?

We may have learned to think of animal products as protein foods. Yet when we look at the balance of calories in many animal products, we see that most calories are from fat. For example, three-quarters of the calories in cheese are from fat, and more than half of the calories in beef or eggs. Apart from the lactose sugar in milk, most animal products lack carbohydrates, which is an essential fuel for the brain. The ways in which foods are described can be misleading. For example, 100 grams of 2 percent milk (reduced-fat milk) contains 2 grams of fat and 89 grams of water. Yet when we look at the balance of calories in 2 percent milk, more than one-third of its calories are from fat (page 39). In whole milk, 48 percent of the calories are from fat. Cow's milk is designed by nature to approximately double the weight of a newborn calf in two months.

While whole plant foods tend to be good protein providers, extracted foods such as sugar or oil can be all carbohydrate or all fat. Natural plant foods provide some carbohydrates, delivered in a way that helps keep our blood sugar level within the normal range. Carbohydrate is the necessary fuel for our brains.

The fat in plant foods is used in cell membranes throughout the body and provides cushioning for our internal organs. When fat comes from whole plant foods, it also delivers fat-soluble vitamins A, E, and K and essential fatty acids. The balance of macronutrients in plant foods has many benefits.

Table 4.1, below, presents the calories and grams of protein in typical servings of various foods. It also shows the balance between the three macronutrients that provide calories: protein, carbohydrate, and fat. Don't be surprised if amounts vary slightly from table to table or online. Weights can vary due to chopping or packing, or the use of metric or imperial measures. Note that in this table we use 1 cup to mean 250 ml, a metric measure. The amounts and balance of the macronutrients can vary with a plant's growing conditions or variety. Also, for packaged foods, see labels. For example, the amount of protein in tofu can vary depending on its firmness and water content.

TABLE 4.1. Calories, protein, and the percentage of calories from protein, carbohydrate, and fat

FOOD	CALORIES PER UNIT, GRAMS	PROTEIN PER UNIT, GRAMS	PERCENT CALORIES FROM PROTEIN	PERCENT CALORIES FROM CARBS	PERCENT CALORIES FROM FAT
LEGUMES AND PRODUCTS					
Adzuki beans, cooked (½ c./122 g)	156	9	23	76	1
Black beans, cooked (½ c./91 g)	120	8	26	70	4
Black-eyed peas, cooked (½ c./90 g)	105	7	26	70	4
Burger, assorted veggie, 1 (71–113 g)*	60–280	7–27	45–65	27–55	6–24
Burger, Awesome, 1 (4 oz./113 g)	280	25	36	13	51
Burger, Beyond, 1 (4 oz/.113 g)	270	20	29	7	64
Burger, Impossible, 1 (4 oz./113 g)	290	27	37	10	53
Chickpeas (garbanzo), cooked (½ c./87 g)	142	8	21	65	14
Cranberry beans, cooked (½ c./94 g)	127	9	27	70	3
Edamame, cooked (½ c./79 g)	106	11	41	36	23
Falafel patties, 3 (2¼ in./51 g)	170	7	16	37	47
Great Northern beans, cooked (½ c./94 g)	110	8	28	69	3
Kidney beans, cooked (½ c./94 g)	119	8	27	70	3
Lentils, cooked (½ c./105 g)	121	9	30	67	3
Lentil sprouts, raw (1 c./81 g)	86	7	28	68	4
Lima beans, cooked (½ c./96 g)	121	8	25	72	3

FOOD	CALORIES PER UNIT, GRAMS	PROTEIN PER UNIT, GRAMS	PERCENT CALORIES FROM PROTEIN	PERCENT CALORIES FROM CARBS	PERCENT CALORIES FROM FAT
Mung beans, cooked (½ c./107 g)	112	7.5	26	71	3
Mung bean sprouts (1 c./110 g)	33	3	33	63	4
Navy beans, cooked (½ c./96 g)	135	8	23	73	4
Pasta, lentil, uncooked (2 oz./56 g)	188–200	11–15	24–25	70–76	0–5
Peanut butter (2 T./32 g)	191–194	7–8	14–16	12–14	71–72
Peanuts (¼ c./37 g)	210	10	17	11	72
Pea sprouts, raw (½ c./63 g)	79	6	24	72	4
Peas, green, raw (½ c./77 g)	62	4	26	70	4
Peas, split, cooked (½ c./104 g)	122	9	27	70	3
Pinto beans, cooked (½ c./90 g)	129	8	25	71	4
Sausage, Beyond, 1 (2.5 oz./76 g)	190	16	33	11	56
Sausage, Field Roast, 1 (3 oz./92 g)	220	25	45	23	32
Soybeans, cooked (½ c./91 g)	156	17	39	18	43
Tempeh, raw (½ c./88 g)*	168	18	39	15	46
Tofu, firm, raw (½ c./133–157 g)*	104–192	12–23	40–44	7–11	49–50
Vegan deli slices (2 oz./60 g)*	72	15	85	14	1
Vegan crumbles, assorted (½ c./53–60 g)*	60–71	10–14	53–71	27–4	0–26
Vegan hot dog, 1 (42–70 g)*	50–163	7–14	26–51	10–15	9–64
White beans/cannellini, cooked (½ c./95 g)	127–137	8–9	27–28	71–72	0–2
NUTS AND SEEDS (raw unless otherwise indicated)					
Almond butter (2 T./32 g)	199	7	13	11	76
Almonds (¼ c./36 g)	209	8	14	14	72
Brazil nut, 1 (5 g)	31	0.7	8	6	86
Brazil nuts (¼ c./34 g)	222	5	8	7	85
Cashew nuts, dry roasted (¼ c./34 g)	199	6	10	21	69
Cashew butter (2 T./32 g)	191	6	11	18	71
Chia seeds, dried (¼ c./43 g)	207	7	13	33	54
Flaxseeds, ground (¼ c./28–32 g)	146–152	5–6	13–14	20–21	65–67
Hazelnuts/filberts (¼ c./34 g)	215	5	9	10	81

FOOD	CALORIES PER UNIT, GRAMS	PROTEIN PER UNIT, GRAMS	PERCENT CALORIES FROM PROTEIN	PERCENT CALORIES FROM CARBS	PERCENT CALORIES FROM FAT
Hemp hearts, hulled (¼ c./41 g)*	224	13	21	6	73
Hemp seeds (¼ c./41 g)*	230	14	24	12	64
Pecans (¼ c./25 g)	173	2	5	7	88
Pine nuts (¼ c./34 g)	201–231	5	7–8	7–11	82–85
Pistachio nuts (¼ c./31 g)	175	6	14	18	68
Poppy seeds (¼ c./34 g)	179	6	13	20	67
Pumpkin seeds (¼ c./33 g)	183	10	20	7	73
Sesame seeds, hulled (¼ c./38 g)	240	8	12	7	81
Sesame seeds, whole (¼ c./37 g)	209	6	12	15	73
Sesame tahini (2 T./30 g)	180	5	11	14	75
Sunflower seed butter (2 T./32 g)	200	6	11	14	75
Sunflower seed kernels (¼ c./36 g)	207	7	13	13	74
Walnuts, black (¼ c./32 g)	196	8	14	6	80
Walnuts, English (¼ c./30 g)	194	5	9	8	83
Water chestnuts, sliced (½ c./66 g)	64	1	5	94	1
GRAINS					
Amaranth, cooked (½ c./130 g)	133	5	14	72	14
Barley, cooked (½ c./83–86 g)	102–104	2	7	90	3
Bread, rye (1 slice/30 g)	78	3	13	75	12
Bread, sprouted Ezekiel (1 slice/30 g)	71	4	20	74	6
Bread, white (1 slice/30 g)*	80	3	14	75	11
Bread, 100% whole wheat (1 slice/30 g)*	71	3	16	74	9
Buckwheat groats, cooked (½ c./89 g)	82	3	13	81	6
Cornmeal, masa harina, cooked (½ c./127 g)	123	3	9	82	9
Corn tortilla, 1 (6 in./26 g)*	58	1	10	80	10
Kamut, cooked (½ c./91 g)	120	5	16	79	5
Millet, cooked (½ c./91 g)	109	3	12	80	8
Oat groats, dry (¼ c./47 g)	183	7	16	69	15
Oats, rolled, dry (¼ c./23 g)	91	4	16	68	16

FOOD	CALORIES PER UNIT, GRAMS	PROTEIN PER UNIT, GRAMS	PERCENT CALORIES FROM PROTEIN	PERCENT CALORIES FROM CARBS	PERCENT CALORIES FROM FAT
Oatmeal, cooked (½ c./124 g)	88	3	14	67	19
Pasta, spaghetti, cooked (½ c./74 g)	117	4	15	80	5
Pasta, whole wheat spaghetti, cooked (½ c./80 g)	119	5	15	75	10
Quinoa, cooked (½ c./98 g)	117	4	15	71	14
Rice, brown, cooked (½ c./103 g)	114–115	2-3	8	85	7
Rice, white, cooked (½ c./84–98 g)	109–128	2	8	91	1
Seitan 1 serving (85 g)*	120	21	66	34	0
Spelt, cooked (½ c./102 g)	130	6	16	78	6
Wheat sprouts (½ c./57 g)	113	4	14	80	5
Wheat tortilla, 1 (6 in./37 g)*	105	3	11	74	15
Wild rice, cooked (½ c./87 g)	88	3	15	82	3
VEGETABLES (raw unless otherwise indicated)					
Arugula, chopped (1 c./21 g)	5	0.6	34	47	19
Asparagus, cooked (½ c./95 g)	21	2	34	59	7
Avocado, sliced (½ c./79 g)	127	2	5	1	76
Beans, snap green/yellow (½ c./53 g)	16	1	20	75	5
Beet greens, chopped, cooked (1 c./40 g)	9	1	32	64	4
Beetroot juice (½ c./125 g)	44	1	12	88	0
Beets, sliced, cooked (½ c./90 g)	40	1.5	14	83	3
Bok choy, shredded (1 c./74 g)	10	1	36	53	11
Broccoli, cooked (½ c./82 g)	29	2	23	68	9
Brussels sprouts, cooked (½ c./82 g)	30	2	24	66	10
Cabbage, green, chopped (1 c./94 g)	24	1	18	79	3
Carrot, chopped, cooked (½ c./82 g)	29	0.6	8	88	4
Carrot, 1 medium (7½ in./61 g)	25	0.6	8	87	5
Carrot juice (½ c./125–127 g)	0	1	9	88	3
Cauliflower, cooked (½ c./66 g)	15	1	26	59	15
Celery, 1 large stalk (11–12 in./64 g)	10	0.4	17	74	9
Collard greens, chopped (1 c./38 g)	12	1	31	55	14

FOOD	CALORIES PER UNIT, GRAMS	PROTEIN PER UNIT, GRAMS	PERCENT CALORIES FROM PROTEIN	PERCENT CALORIES FROM CARBS	PERCENT CALORIES FROM FAT
Corn, yellow/white (½ c./81 g)	70	3	13	75	12
Cucumber, sliced (½ c./55 g)	8	0.4	14	80	6
Eggplant, cubed, cooked (½ c./52 g)	18	0.4	8	87	5
Garlic cloves (2 T./17 g)	26	1	16	81	3
Kale, chopped (1 c./21 g)	10	0.9	28	58	14
Kelp, raw (½ c./42 g)	18	0.7	13	77	10
Leeks, chopped (½ c./47 g)	29	0.7	9	87	4
Lettuce, butterhead, chopped (1 c./58 g)	8	0.8	33	55	12
Lettuce, romaine, chopped (1 c./50 g)	8	0.6	24	63	13
Mushrooms (½ c./44 g)	10	1	37	60	3
Mushrooms, shiitake, 4 (76 g)	26	2	22	67	11
Mustard greens, chopped (1 c./59 g)	16	2	34	55	11
Okra, chopped, cooked (½ c./85 g)	19	2	27	66	7
Onions, green/spring, chopped (½ c./53 g)	17	1	19	77	4
Onions, red/yellow/white, chopped (½ c./85 g)	34	1	10	88	2
Parsnips, cooked (½ c./82 g)	59	1	7	89	4
Peas, fresh (½ c./77 g)	62	4	26	70	4
Pea pods, snow/edible (1 c./67 g)	28	2	26	70	4
Pepper, bell, green, chopped (½ c./79 g)	16	0.7	15	79	6
Pepper, bell, red, chopped (½ c./79 g)	24	0.8	13	78	9
Potato, baked, 1 medium (3 in./173 g)	161	4	10	88	1
Potato, peeled, diced, boiled (½ c./82 g)	71	1	8	91	1
Radishes, sliced (¼ c./29 g)	5	0.2	16	79	5
Rutabaga, chopped, cooked (½ c./90 g)	27	0.8	11	84	5
Spinach, chopped (1 c./32 g)	7	0.9	39	49	12
Spirulina seaweed, dried (1 t./2.3 g)	7	1	58	24	18
Squash, acorn, cubed, baked (½ c./108 g)	61	1	7	91	2
Squash, butternut, cubed, baked (½ c./108 g)	43	1	8	90	2
Squash, hubbard, baked (½ c./108 g)	54	3	17	74	9

FOOD	CALORIES PER UNIT, GRAMS	PROTEIN PER UNIT, GRAMS	PERCENT CALORIES FROM PROTEIN	PERCENT CALORIES FROM CARBS	PERCENT CALORIES FROM FAT
Squash, summer, cooked (½ c./95 g)	19	0.9	15	73	12
Sweet potato, peeled, baked (½ c./106 g)	95	2	9	90	1
Tomato, chopped (½ c./95 g)	17	0.9	17	74	9
Tomato, 1 medium (2 in./123 g)	22	1	17	74	9
Turnip, chopped, boiled (½ c./82 g)	18	0.6	12	85	3
Turnip greens, chopped (1 c./58 g)	19	0.9	16	77	7
Watercress greens, chopped (1 c./36 g)	4	0.8	60	34	6
Yam, peeled, baked (½ c./105 g)	95	2	9	90	1
Zucchini, chopped (½ c./66 g)	11	0.8	24	62	14
FRUITS (fresh unless indicated)					
Apple 1 medium (182 g)	95	0.5	2	95	3
Apricot 1 medium (35 g)	17	0.5	10	83	7
Apricots, dried (¼ c./33 g)	79–82	1	4–5	93–96	0–2
Banana, 1 medium (118 g)	105	1	4	93	3
Blackberries (½ c./76 g)	33	1	12	79	9
Blueberries (½ c./78 g)	45	0.6	4	91	5
Cantaloupe, diced (½ c./82 g)	28	0.7	9	87	4
Cherries (½ c./81 g)	51	0.9	6	91	3
Coconut, dried, unsweetened (¼ c./20 g)	134	1	4	13	83
Cranberries (½ c./53 g)	24	0.2	4	94	2
Currants, dried (¼ c./37 g)	103	1.5	5	94	1
Dates, pitted (¼ c./37 g)	102–105	0.7–0.9	2–3	96–97	1
Durian, chopped (½ c./128 g)	189	2	4	67	29
Fig, 1 medium (2¼ in./50 g)	37	0.4	4	93	3
Figs, dried (¼ c./38 g)	94	1	5	92	3
Grapefruit, 1 medium (3¾ in./246 g)	103	2	7	90	3
Grapes (½ c./80 g)	55	0.6	4	94	2
Guava (½ c./87 g)	59	2	14	75	11
Honeydew melon, diced (½ c./90 g)	32	0.5	6	91	3

FOOD	CALORIES PER UNIT, GRAMS	PROTEIN PER UNIT, GRAMS	PERCENT CALORIES FROM PROTEIN	PERCENT CALORIES FROM CARBS	PERCENT CALORIES FROM FAT
Kiwifruit, 1 medium, (2 in./150 g)	42	0.8	7	86	7
Kiwifruit, sliced (½ c./95 g)	58	1	7	86	7
Mango, 1 medium (2 in./131 g)	202	3	5	90	5
Orange, 1 medium (2 in./150 g)	62	1	7	91	2
Orange juice (½ c./131 g)	59	0.9	6	90	4
Papaya, chopped (½ c./77 g)	33	0.4	4	91	5
Peach, 1 medium (2 in./150 g)	58	1	8	87	5
Pear, 1 medium (178 g)	101	0.6	2	96	2
Pineapple, diced (½ c./87 g)	44	0.5	4	94	2
Plum, 1 medium (66 g)	30	0.5	5	90	5
Prunes, pitted (¼ c./44 g)	106	1	3	96	1
Raisins (¼ c., packed/42 g)	125	1	4	95	1
Raspberries (½ c./65 g)	34	0.8	8	82	10
Strawberries (½ c./76 g)	24	0.5	7	85	8
Watermelon, diced (½ c./80 g)	24	0.5	7	89	4
NONDAIRY BEVERAGES (unsweetened)*					
Almond milk (1 c./250 ml)	42	2	16	16	68
Hemp milk (1 c./250 ml)	63–85	2–3	9–23	0–5	77–86
Oat milk (1 c./250 g)	50	1	8	48	44
Pea milk (1 c./250 ml)	80	8	42	4	54
Rice milk (1 c./250 ml)	119	0.7	2	79	19
Soy milk (1 c./250 ml)	74–127	7–13	32–40	17–27	41–44
OILS, FATS, AND SWEETENERS					
Maple syrup (1 T./20 g)	53	0	0	100	0
Margarine (1 T./14 g)*	101	0	0	0	100
Oil: avocado, canola, coconut, flaxseed, olive (1 T./14 g)*	121–126	0	0	0	100
Sugar (1 T./12 g)	49	0	0	100	0

FOOD	CALORIES PER UNIT, GRAMS	PROTEIN PER UNIT, GRAMS	PERCENT CALORIES FROM PROTEIN	PERCENT CALORIES FROM CARBS	PERCENT CALORIES FROM FAT
ANIMAL PRODUCTS (uncooked)					
Beef, ground, 20% fat, 80% lean (3 oz./90 g)	229	16	28	0	72
Beef, ground, 10% fat, 90% lean (3 oz./90 g)	158	18	47	0	53
Cheddar cheese, medium (1 oz./30 g)*	121	7	23	3	74
Chicken breast (3 oz./90 g)	154	19	50	0	50
Cow's milk, 2% (1 c./258 g)	129	8	26	38**	36
Egg, 1 large (50 g)	72	6	36	2	62
Salmon, Atlantic coho, farmed (3 oz./90 g)	144–187	18–19	40–55	0	45–60
Salmon, Atlantic coho, wild (3 oz./90 g)	128–131	18–19	58–62	0	38–42

KEY: 1 tablespoon = 15 ml, ¼ cup = 60 ml, ½ cup = 125 ml, 1 cup = 250 ml • c. = cup, T. = tablespoon, t. = teaspoon, oz. = ounce, in. = inch, g = gram, ml = milliliter

Sources: US Department of Agriculture (fdc.nal.usda.gov) and ESHA Research (esha.com/products/food-processor).

*Check package labels for brand-specific amounts.

**Lactose sugar

Answers to the quiz on page 31

1. Arugula, asparagus, bok choy, butterhead or red leaf lettuce, mushrooms, mustard greens, napa (Chinese) cabbage, and spinach
2. 90 percent lean ground beef, chicken breast, egg, and salmon
3. Beef, even "lean" beef (which is 10 percent fat by weight, but 53 percent of the calories are from fat), cheddar cheese, chicken breast, egg, and salmon
4. Plant-based meat alternatives (such as burgers, sausages, veggie deli slices), edamame, tofu, and seitan
5. Peanuts, peanut butter, Beyond Sausage, nuts, seeds, nut and seed butters, avocado, almond milk, hemp milk, pea milk, and oils
6. The highest-protein fruits are apricots, blackberries, cantaloupe, and guava. Fruits provide less protein than foods in other plant-based food groups, and most provide 2–8 percent of calories from protein.

References for this chapter are online at https://plant-poweredprotein.com/references.

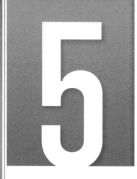

The Environmental Costs of Protein Choices

Our lives depend on the environment: the air we breathe, the water we drink, and the land we call home. This chapter explores the relationship between the food we eat and our environment. It demonstrates that as individuals, we have the power to effect change by choosing to spend money in ways that stimulate our economies, support communities, and promote environmental stewardship.

THE CLIMATE CRISIS

The climate crisis can be so intense that it leaves us feeling powerless. It's no wonder that some people remain willfully ignorant, while others are plagued by guilt when their actions do not align with their values. It is tempting to offset our responsibility by blaming industry or government. But the truth is that industry is driven by our choices and governments by our votes. Supply and demand start with you and me. We cast our votes with every dollar we spend and every politician we elect.

Predictions about catastrophic future events linked to climate change loom large. Yet it is no longer reasonable to talk about climate change as "future events" because it's a crisis now. Its impact on our economy, infrastructure, human health, and ecosystems cannot be ignored. According to NASA, the average global temperature has increased by 2.12 degrees F (1.18 degrees C) since the late 19th century, largely as a result of human activity.

Why be concerned about a few degrees? A small shift in average temperature creates new weather extremes. What were viewed as "extremes" are now common with stronger and more intense hurricanes, droughts, floods, and wildfires. Such events threaten water resources, agriculture, power supplies, wildlife, and infrastructure. We must also consider the economic burden imposed when funds required for social welfare, education, medicine, technology, and science are diverted to climate events.

Experts predict that from 2021 to 2026, climate change, deforestation, and water insecurity will cost businesses $1.26 trillion internationally. Just in the past decade, American taxpayers spent more than $350 billion to address climate crisis events. Swiss Re Group, one of the world's largest insurance companies, reported that climate change could result in a global decline in productivity of $23 trillion by 2050. If we act now, much of this cost could be reduced. The United Nations Environment Programme asserts that if the United States invested $1.8 trillion to address climate change, it would return $7.1 trillion in avoided costs, among other benefits.

With all the discourse on climate change, impacts of agriculture are often underrepresented. Below, we will show how dietary choices can be one of the most effective ways we can reduce our carbon footprint.

Animal agriculture is a major driver of climate change. Estimates for the total percentage of greenhouse gas (GHG) emissions that are linked to animal agriculture range widely. Some experts claim that estimates at the lower end of this range fail to include all emission sources and assign some emissions to the wrong sectors. One often-referenced estimate was published by the United Nations' Food and Agriculture Organization (FAO) in 2013. It suggested that animal agriculture is responsible for 14.5 percent of total GHG emissions. This was slightly lower than its 2006 estimate of 18 percent. A Worldwatch Institute report criticized the FAO's 18 percent estimate, alleging that the FAO overlooked or underreported livestock respiration, land use change, and methane production, among other factors. The Worldwatch Institute concluded that when these are considered, animal agriculture accounts for at least 51 percent of total GHGs. Several reports have since criticized the FAO's findings, providing alternative estimates from 16.5 percent to 87 percent.

Estimating the total GHGs from animal agriculture is clearly a difficult and complex task. Wherever on the spectrum the total lies, experts tend to agree that it is a significant contributor to climate change. Shifting the dietary patterns of populations must be a priority for policymakers if we are to stand any chance of mitigating its effects.

Let's compare the GHG emissions from a variety of protein sources. Figure 5.1 (page 42) shows the average GHG emissions by food product based on some of the most comprehensive research on this topic.

It is indisputable that animal products are significantly more carbon intensive than plant foods. When coauthor Cory Davis was completing his bachelor's degree, his biochemistry professor asked the class to use a carbon footprint calculator. Several students biked to school each day. Cory drove most days due to his distance from school. Regardless, his carbon footprint was the lowest in the class. The cyclists in class protested, saying, "But we bike and he drives. How could his carbon footprint be lower than ours?" The teacher looked at Cory, and the class, and replied: "He doesn't eat meat."

The bottom line is that our food choices are a powerful personal tool for reducing our carbon footprint. We need one simple dietary shift—more plants, less

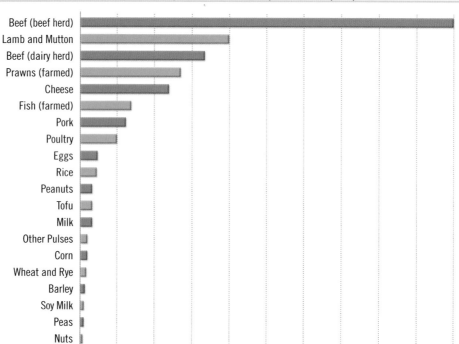

FIGURE 5.1. GHG emissions (pounds of CO_2 equivalents) per pound of food.

Source: Poore J, Nemecek T. "Reducing food's environmental impacts through producers and consumers," *Science* 360, no. 6392 (June 1, 2018): 987–992.

meat. Compare beef with tofu. Beef, on average, creates more than 31 times more GHG emissions per kilogram than tofu. Even poultry, the least carbon-intensive meat, creates more than three times the emissions. Other legumes leave an even softer footprint than tofu. Compare beef with beans, shown as "other pulses" in figure 5.1, above. Per kilogram, beef emits more than 55 times more GHG emissions than beans, and poultry emits more than five times more.

The impacts of our changing climate go far beyond their damage to fragile ecosystems. They have profound political, social, and economic repercussions. These impacts are not equally distributed. In any country, the effects of climate change are absorbed disproportionately by Indigenous populations, minorities, and the poor. Disadvantaged groups tend to live in areas that are more exposed to climate hazards and susceptible to damages. This inequality reduces their ability to cope with and recover from these onslaughts. Countries that emit high levels of GHGs export the damage they create to more vulnerable countries. In fact, 20 of the 36 countries with the highest GHG emissions are among the least impacted by climate change. Of the 17 countries producing the lowest emissions, 11 are the most impacted. There are inequalities in age and gender as well. In many susceptible nations, women are responsible for firewood and water collection, making them more vulnerable to climate hazards. The young and the old are less protected, as they are more fragile and less mobile. If we are concerned with social justice, being mindful of our carbon "food-prints" can be a powerful tool to support people who are less privileged.

Agriculture subsidies are a matter of social justice. Subsidies on meat, dairy, and animal feed drives their prices down, artificially reducing international prices. Lower prices raise demand, resulting in more emissions. This effect is so potent that poorer countries, which cannot afford significant subsidies, must import food that local farmers could have grown more efficiently. Local farmers may exit the market entirely, as they cannot compete. According to the FAO, if the United States alone were to stop subsidizing agriculture, where most subsidies go toward animal agriculture, it would lift millions out of poverty around the world. (See pages 3–4 for more on subsidies.)

LAND USE AND GLOBAL FOOD SECURITY

H alf of all habitable land on planet Earth is used for agriculture. Yes, half. This leaves only 37 percent for forests, 11 percent for shrub ecosystems, 1 percent for fresh water, and 1 percent for urban development. Although most of the agricultural land is used for meat and dairy production, this accounts for only 17 percent of calories produced. The United States claims to produce the world's most sustainable meat. Yet, if the entire global population ate the average American diet, we would need to convert 100 percent of the planet's habitable land into agricultural land, and we would still fall almost 40 percent short.

Land use poses complex challenges for future food security. Each ecosystem is unique and the rising demand for animal products impacts regions differently. Where pasture or grasslands do not exist, forests are being destroyed to make them. Deforestation is occurring at a staggering rate. From 1990 to 2020, approximately 1.037 billion acres (420 million hectares) of forest were lost. Agriculture is the primary driver of deforestation globally. In the tropics, pasture expansion for livestock leads to the loss of more than 5 million acres (2 million hectares) of forest per year. This does not include expansion of cropland for animal feed. In the United States, where per capita meat intakes are among the highest in the world, most of the beef produced is consumed domestically. Where demand for beef is increasing, it is often imported from countries such as Brazil, the foremost example of livestock-driven deforestation.

Some argue that using pasture for livestock is an efficient means of producing food. There is, after all, much more "pasture" than cropland. Natural pastures are grasslands, many of which are essential ecosystems for a wide range of species. However, few livestock graze their entire lives. In the United States, less than 1 percent of cattle are "grass finished," which means raised entirely on pasture. This is not to be confused with "grass fed," which applies to almost all cattle, which graze at some stage. Contrary to what you might imagine, grass-finished cattle produce even more GHG emissions than feedlot cattle. This is because they reach market weight more slowly and more methane is produced digesting grass. Typically, cattle graze for most of their first year. Then they are sent to the feedlot where they are fed grains and legumes for finishing. Farmer associations often recommend preparing cattle for the feedlot diet. This is done by "creep feeding," or slowly introducing grains into their diet to increase their acceptance of feedlot fare. Feedlots make cattle economically feasible by driving weight gain by about three pounds per day. This makes them more valuable. They are fattened for 60 to 200 days before slaughter. So, even though cows use "pasture," the vast majority rely on cropland for feed. In fact, only about 55 percent of the world's cropland, the highest-value agricultural land, is used to feed humans directly. About 9 percent is used for biofuels and industry while 36 percent is dedicated to animal fodder. In the United States, where animal products are in high demand, more than half of the grains grown on cropland are used for animal feed. Livestock are so inefficient at converting calories that if we were to redirect crops used for animal feed and biofuels to humans, we could increase the calorie production globally by as much as 70 percent, enough to feed an additional four billion people. Even slight shifts in the use of our cropland to feed humans directly could wipe out hunger, if done thoughtfully.

How much land, including pasture, do different food sources require? Let's take a look at figure 5.2 (page 45).

As you can see, lamb, mutton, and beef require the most land by far. Non-dairy cattle on average use 1,592 square feet of land to produce 1 pound of product. Tofu, by comparison, only uses 17 square feet for 1 pound of product. Beef requires more than 93 times more land than tofu per kilogram of food.

Meat enthusiasts argue that vegan claims about land use by cattle are exaggerated. They point out that cattle use much more pasture than arable cropland. They are correct. Approximately 86.8 percent of the land cattle use is pasture and only 13.2 percent is cropland. Using these numbers, more than 210 square feet of cropland is required per pound of beef. By these estimates, beef uses over 12 times more cropland than tofu. In other words, we could produce more than 12 pounds of tofu for every 1 pound of beef with the same amount of cropland. But natural pastures are grasslands, many of which are fragile and/or critically important ecosystems. These ecosystems provide soil and water conservation, pollination, climate regulation, and essential habitat for many species, including species at risk. Furthermore, many pastures have been artifically developed by

FIGURE 5.2. Land use (square feet) per pound of food produced.

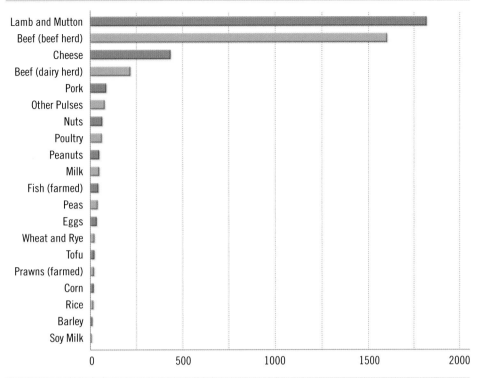

Source: Poore J, Nemecek T. "Reducing food's environmental impacts through producers and consumers," *Science* 360, no. 6392 (June 1, 2018): 987–992.

expansion into forests and other ecosystems. Each year, this results in a global loss of more than 5 million acres (2 million hectares) of forest.

WATER CONSUMPTION

I f you have ever lived through a drought, you are aware of the challenges that lack of water can impose on communities. With climate change, combined droughts and heatwaves are becoming more frequent. Blame for water scarcity is often directed at the oil and gas industry, bottled water companies, or irresponsible personal water use, such as excessive watering of lawns and long showers. While these consume water, what we choose to eat can have an even more dramatic impact.

Water is essential for life, playing a critical role in all ecosystems. It is replenished through the water cycle, evaporating from the oceans and returning via rain to our lakes and rivers. We use fresh water for drinking, hydroelectric dams, irrigation, and industrial purposes. Only 2.5 percent of our water resources consist of fresh water. About 70 percent of this is locked up in glaciers and snow. Water is unequally distributed, as over 2.3 billion people live in regions where water is scarce.

Agriculture is the largest user of this precious resource, requiring 70 to 85 percent of the total demand. Environmental activists often target activities like fracking, a process of procuring oil and gas from shale rock that uses 70–140 billion gallons of water annually. Yet agriculture uses tens of trillions of gallons of water annually. Perhaps because it is necessary for life, water lacks economic valuation as an agricultural asset. Oil, for example, is treated as a commodity and traded in the marketplace for revenue. Often, agricultural users pay little or nothing for water withdrawal. As a result, the prices of agricultural products don't reflect the true cost of their water requirements, and incentives to reduce its use are lacking.

We have been told to be frugal about our water usage at home. Yet our home water use makes up only about 4 percent of total human water consumption. The rest lies in the things we purchase from industries like oil and gas, chemicals, smelting, manufacturing, and the largest user, agriculture. If you are concerned about water scarcity and reducing your water footprint, your most powerful action is to reduce your consumption of water-intensive foods.

How much fresh water do our food choices consume? As figure 5.3 (page 47) shows, cheese and nuts require the most water per pound. Some may use this information to point a finger at nut-eating vegans. While the figures are accurate, remember that a pound is a whole lot of nuts. One serving of nuts is an ounce (less than 30 g). Thus, a pound provides 16 servings. Meat is consumed in larger amounts, often 4 ounces (113 g) and sometimes more. Compared to 16 servings of nuts, a pound of 4-ounce steaks yields 4 servings. If we look at the figures per 100 calories, pork, dairy herd beef, and milk all require more water than nuts. (Note that after their milk production drops at about age six, dairy cows are made into burger meat.) The current health recommendation is to replace meat with a wide variety of legumes, such as beans, peas, chickpeas, lentils, and tofu, plus a limited amount of nuts. Per serving, farmed fish and prawns are the most water-intensive, animal-derived protein sources, followed by beef from dairy cattle, lamb, pork, and beef from beef cattle. The most water-intensive, plant-based protein sources are nuts, rice, and peanuts.

So, let's do the math. Beef from beef cattle, a less water-intensive animal product, requires 173.9 gallons of fresh water per pound of final product. Tofu requires 17.8 gallons. Therefore, beef requires almost 10 times more water than tofu. Dairy cattle require less land than beef cattle but need far more water—325.2 gallons per pound or 18 times more than tofu. Poultry, often considered a healthier and more environmentally friendly alternative to beef, requires 79.1 gallons of water per pound, more than four times that of tofu.

FIGURE 5.3. Fresh water consumption in gallons per pound of food.

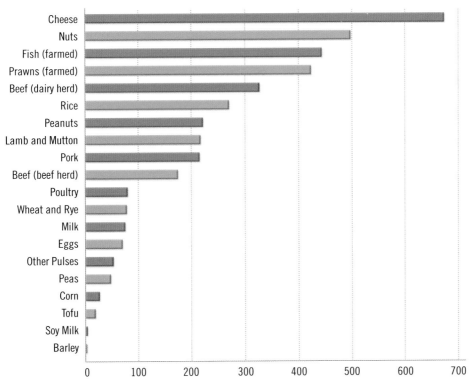

Source: Poore J, Nemecek T. "Reducing food's environmental impacts through producers and consumers," *Science* 360, no. 6392 (June 1, 2018): 987–992.

We have compared meat with tofu several times during this discourse. Meat advocates often point out that most soybean crops are often genetically modified (GMO), use lots of pesticides, and operate with massive monocultures. For example, the *Sacred Cow* documentary website asserted that "proponents of plant-based protein also fail to address how our current monoculture systems of intensive corn and soybean production have caused a number of environmental challenges." Critical points omitted from their assertion include:

1. Large GMO plantations, many of which spray crops with hazardous pesticides, account for 94 percent of soybean production. Most of this is used for animal feed.

2. Soybean production for human consumption is 7 percent. Of that, the lion's share goes into soybean oil and processed foods. Tofu for human consumption in most of the Western world is almost always from GMO-free soybeans.

3. Animal feed accounts for 77 percent of soybean production (over three-quarters of soy grown worldwide and more than 70 percent in the United States). Animal-feed production drives the demand for pesticides in these large monocultures.

4. The remainder of soy production is destined for industrial purposes, such as lubricants and biofuels.

We can see the criticisms of soy are mainly connected with the meat industry. Plant-based eaters consume mostly non-GMO soy directly, while meat eaters consume GMO soy indirectly. Nearly half of all the corn grown in the United States goes to domestic animal feed; 11 percent is exported, primarily for animal feed in other countries. About 30 percent goes to ethanol production. Less than 8 percent is for human consumption, and much of that is for high-fructose corn syrup. These vast monocultures of soy and corn are strongly linked with the animal-products industry.

In short, by minimizing animal products and expanding our diets to include a wide variety of plants, we can greatly reduce pressure on our dwindling water resources. For more sustainable management of these resources, plant-based diets are a leap in the right direction.

WATER QUALITY

Water pollution is a global issue that affects economic growth and the health of billions. Agriculture plays a major role by releasing large amounts of pesticides, fertilizers, drug residues, and sediments into our bodies of water. This increases the risk to ecosystems, drinking water, and economic potential. Almost 40 percent of the water bodies in the European Union are significantly harmed by agricultural pollution. In the United States, agriculture is the largest polluter of rivers and streams and a significant polluter of wetlands and lakes. Livestock operations are growing fast, increasing the quantities of waste manure, pesticides, and fertilizers. New pollutants have emerged from this industry over the past few decades. These come in the form of antibiotics, vaccines, and growth hormones that enter ecosystems and drinking water. The World Health Organization recognizes pathogens from animal waste in water as an important health concern.

Animal products dominate the top of the water pollution list (high impact), while plant products dominate the bottom half (low impact). Compare beef from beef cattle, which has less impact than dairy cattle, and tofu. Beef emits around 4.82 ounces of water pollution per pound of beef. Tofu emits just 0.1 ounce of pollution per pound. It would take roughly 48 pounds of

FIGURE 5.4. Water pollution in ounces of phosphate equivalents per pound of product.

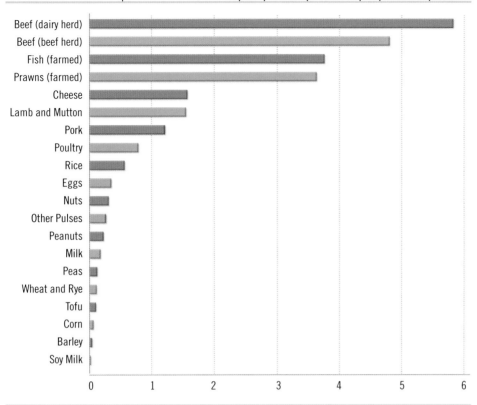

Source: Poore J, Nemecek T. "Reducing food's environmental impacts through producers and consumers," *Science* 360, no. 6392 (June 1, 2018): 987–992.

tofu to create the same impact on water quality as 1 pound of beef. Farmed fish also has a high impact, at around 3.63 ounces of pollution per pound. It would take around 36 pounds of tofu to match that same level of water pollution. Poultry has the lowest impact among the meats, producing around 0.78 ounce of pollution per pound. Still, it would take 7.8 pounds of tofu to match the impact of one pound of poultry.

Agriculture, especially animal agriculture, is responsible for a large portion of our water-quality challenges. Replacing animal products with plant-based alternatives such as tofu is a wise move. Again, choosing plant protein is an effective way to mitigate the environmental impacts of agriculture.

There is no question that intensive animal agriculture poses a massive and unnecessary environmental burden. It's a notorious polluter and among the greatest contributors to deforestation, desertification, and species extinction.

Policymakers must take action. We need to recognize that while animal agriculture continues to be subsidized, we are paying the price with our planet. Shifting toward a plant-based food economy is no longer an option; it is an ecological imperative. Making this dietary shift may well be one of the most powerful steps any individual can take toward the preservation of life on earth. Together we can make a monumental difference and pave the way to a more compassionate, ethical, and environmentally responsible future for humanity. It starts with you and me, here and now.

References for this chapter are online at https://plant-poweredprotein.com/references.

Protein in Health and Disease

When it comes to health and disease, protein matters because not getting enough can harm our ability to build and repair body tissues. Yet certain protein sources can increase our risk of disease. To promote health and prevent disease, we need enough protein from healthful food sources. For most people, getting enough protein is easy. Many Americans get double the protein they need. People eating 100 percent plant-based diets generally meet or exceed protein needs. People who fall short may not be eating enough calories or an adequate variety of foods.

While avoiding nutritional shortfalls is important, avoiding excesses is too. Globally, while close to a billion people suffer from undernutrition or hunger, almost twice as many suffer from diseases of nutritional excess, such as obesity and type 2 diabetes. Diet-induced chronic diseases are responsible for about 70 percent of deaths worldwide. This means that any question of food quality must factor in the impact of that food on disease risk.

This chapter explores the relationship between protein sources, mortality, and the risk of common chronic diseases. We conclude with an examination of the key reasons why plant protein provides a solid health advantage.

PROTEIN SOURCES AND MORTALITY

We often hear that generous protein intakes offer protection as we age. Higher protein intakes help to preserve muscle mass, reduce falls, improve bone strength, and decrease the risk of fractures. But all protein sources aren't equal. When it comes to mortality (death rate), the weight of evidence suggests that the source of protein matters. People who get their protein from plants enjoy a distinct advantage over those who get their protein from animals.

Jaw Droppers

STUDY 1: United States, 416,104 participants (Huang, 2020)

- Drop in overall mortality when 3 percent of calories from animal protein are replaced with plant protein: 10 percent
- Drop in mortality when 3 percent of calories from dairy products are replaced with plant protein: 8 percent
- Drop in mortality when 3 percent of calories from red meat are replaced with plant protein: 13 percent for men, 15 percent for women
- Drop in mortality when 3 percent of calories from egg protein are replaced with plant protein: 2 percent for men, 21 percent for women

STUDY 2: China, Meta-analysis of 12 studies, 483,615 participants (Qi, 2020)

- Drop in total mortality per 3 percent increase in plant protein intake: 3 percent
- Increase in total mortality per 3 percent increase in animal protein intake: 5 percent

STUDY 3: Iran, 715,128 participants (Naghshi, 2020)

- Drop in overall mortality with the addition of 3 percent of calories from plant protein: 5 percent

STUDY 4: Japan, 70,696 participants (Budhathoki, 2019)

- Drop in total mortality when 3 percent of calories from red meat are replaced with plant protein: 34 percent
- Drop in total mortality when 3 percent of calories from processed meat are replaced with plant protein: 46 percent

STUDY 5: United States, 15,428 participants (Seidelmann, 2018)

- Increase in mortality when carbohydrates are replaced with animal-derived fat or protein: 18 percent*
- Drop in mortality when carbohydrates are replaced with plant-derived fat or protein: 18 percent*

*Carbohydrates in these populations were mostly refined or of poor quality.

STUDY 6: United States, 262,684 participants (Song, 2016)

- Increase in mortality when 3 percent of calories from plant protein are replaced by 3 percent of calories as protein from unprocessed red meat: 12 percent

- Increase in mortality when 3 percent of calories from plant protein are replaced by 3 percent of calories as protein from eggs: 19 percent
- Rise in mortality when 3 percent of calories from plant protein are replaced by 3 percent of calories as protein from processed red meat: 34 percent

STUDY 7: United States, 6,381 participants (Levine, 2014)

- Increase in all-cause mortality in people aged 50–65 who consume a high-protein diet (20 percent or more of calories from protein): 74 percent*

  *These associations were eliminated or diminished if the proteins were plant derived.

PROTEIN SOURCES AND CARDIOVASCULAR DISEASE

What foods are most strongly implicated in cardiovascular disease (CVD)? There is no question that meat, especially red and processed meat, is implicated. Regardless, low carbohydrate proponents claim that it is not meat, but rather carbohydrate that is the real killer. Their thinking is that hamburgers may be guilty as charged, but the guilt lies with the bun not the beef. While there is solid evidence against refined carbohydrates (e.g., sugar and white flour products), unrefined carbohydrates (e.g., carbohydrates that are intrinsic to whole plant foods) are proven protective. The evidence on CVD outcomes with varying intakes of animal and plant protein is clear and consistent. Animal protein, especially from red and processed meat, increases our risk of CVD, while plant protein reduces risk.

Jaw Droppers

STUDY 1: United States, 29,682 participants (Zhong, 2020)

- Increase in cardiovascular disease risk with two versus zero servings of unprocessed meat per week: 4 percent*
- Increase in cardiovascular disease risk with two versus zero servings of processed meat per week: 11 percent**

  *1 serving = 4 ounces/113 g
  **1 serving = 2 slices bacon (½ oz./14 g), 1 wiener (1¼ oz./35 g)

STUDY 2: China, 483,615 participants (Qi, 2020)

- Increase in cardiovascular disease risk comparing highest versus lowest intake of animal protein: 11 percent

- Drop in cardiovascular disease risk comparing highest versus lowest intake of plant protein: 8 percent

STUDY 3: United States, 456 participants (Razavi, 2020)
- Increase in early heart failure risk in the highest versus lowest tertile (33.3 percent of group) of animal-protein intake: 251 percent
- Increase in early heart failure risk in the highest versus lowest tertile of processed-meat intake: 200 percent
- Drop in early heart failure risk in the highest versus lowest tertile of whole-grain intake: 9 percent
- Drop in early heart failure risk in the highest versus lowest tertile of fresh-vegetable intake: 53 percent
- Drop in early heart failure risk in the highest versus lowest tertile of legume intake: 56 percent

STUDY 4: United States, 81,337 participants in Adventist Health Study-2 cohort (Tharrey, 2018)
- Increase in cardiovascular disease mortality for each 0.6 ounce (18 g) of daily animal-protein intake: 12 percent
- Drop in cardiovascular disease mortality for each 0.6 ounce (18 g) of daily plant-protein intake: 5 percent
- Increase in cardiovascular disease mortality in the highest versus lowest quintile (20 percent of group) of meat intake: 67 percent
- Drop in cardiovascular disease mortality in the highest versus lowest quintile of nut and seed intake: 41 percent

STUDY 5: China, 2,079,236 participants (Yang, 2016)
- Increase in total stroke risk comparing highest versus lowest total red-meat intake: 14 percent*
- Increase in total stroke risk comparing highest versus lowest processed meat intake: 17 percent*
- Increase in ischemic stroke risk comparing highest versus lowest total red-meat intake: 22 percent
- Intake of red meat that significantly increased risk for total stroke: 2.5 ounces (70 g) per day
- Intake of processed meat that significantly increased risk for total stroke: any amount more than 0 grams per day

*Total stroke refers to both ischemic and hemorrhagic stroke.

PROTEIN SOURCES AND TYPE 2 DIABETES

Many popular diets used to prevent or treat type 2 diabetes are low-carbohydrate diets, and, as such, contain generous amounts of animal protein. Meat is emphasized because it is carbohydrate-free. Even though it may sound reasonable to chow down on low-carbohydrate foods if you want to rid yourself of type 2 diabetes, it takes more than being carbohydrate-free. After protein, the remaining calories in meat come from fat. In "lean" beef, 53 percent of calories come from fat (see page 39). Much of that is saturated fat, which can increase insulin resistance and LDL cholesterol. When you look at the evidence, meat fails to measure up to hopes. Studies consistently report higher rates of type 2 diabetes with higher meat intakes. The strongest associations are for processed meat and red meat. By contrast, foods rich in plant protein have proven to be protective.

Jaw Droppers

STUDY 1: Netherlands, 6,822 participants (Chen, 2020)

- Increase in risk of prediabetes per 5 percent increment of energy from animal protein at the expense of carbohydrate: 35 percent
- Increase in risk of type 2 diabetes per 5 percent increment of energy from animal protein at the expense of carbohydrate: 37 percent

STUDY 2: Finland, 2,332 male participants (Virtanen, 2017)

- Increase in type 2 diabetes risk by replacing 1 percent of calories from carbohydrates with protein: 5 percent
- Drop in type 2 diabetes risk by replacing 1 percent of calories from animal protein with plant protein: 18 percent

STUDY 3: China, meta-analysis, 11 studies, 483,174 participants (Tian, 2017)

- Increase in type 2 diabetes risk for highest versus lowest intake of animal protein: 14 percent
- Drop in type 2 diabetes risk for highest versus lowest intake of plant protein: 4 percent
- Increase in type 2 diabetes risk for highest versus lowest intake of red meat: 22 percent
- Increase in type 2 diabetes risk for highest versus lowest intake of processed meat: 39 percent
- Drop in type 2 diabetes risk for highest versus lowest intake of soy: 26 percent

STUDY 4: United States, 205,802 participants (Malik, 2016)

- Increase in type 2 diabetes risk in the highest versus lowest quintile (20 percent of group) of animal protein intake: 13 percent

- Drop in type 2 diabetes risk in the highest versus lowest quintile of plant protein intake: 9 percent

- Drop in type 2 diabetes risk by replacing 5 percent of calories from animal protein with plant protein: 23 percent

STUDY 5: United States, 6,381 (Levine, 2014)

- Increase in type 2 diabetes mortality in people aged 50–65 with high protein intake (20 percent or more of calories): 393 percent (almost four times)*

- Increase in type 2 diabetes mortality in people aged 66 or older with high protein intake (20 percent or more of calories): 1,064 percent (more than 10 times)*

  *Compared to people with low-protein intake (less than 10 percent of calories)

PROTEIN SOURCES AND CANCER

One of the strongest associations we have for meat and chronic disease risk is colorectal cancer. Both processed meat and red meat are implicated. The World Health Organization has declared processed meat a Group 1 or *convincing* human carcinogen. Red meat is categorized as a Group 2A or *probable* human carcinogen. This means there is convincing evidence that processed meat causes cancer and limited evidence that red meat causes cancer. Even small amounts of processed meat, such as cold cuts, bacon, ham, sausage, pepperoni, wieners, and bologna, can increase the risk of colorectal cancer. According to the American Institute for Cancer Research, daily consumption of 1.8 ounces (50 g) of processed meat, such as one wiener, increases colorectal cancer risk by about 16 percent.

Jaw Droppers

STUDY 1: Iran, Meta-analysis of 23 studies, 330,826 participants (Nachvak, 2020)

- Drop in total cancer risk with each increase of 10 milligrams per day of soy isoflavone intake: 7 percent

- Drop in breast cancer risk with each increase of 10 milligrams per day of soy isoflavone intake: 9 percent

- Drop in breast cancer death with each 0.18 ounce (5 g) per day of soy protein intake: 12 percent

STUDY 2: Japan, 70,696 participants (Budhathoki, 2019)

- Drop in cancer-related mortality when 3 percent of calories from red meat are replaced with plant protein: 39 percent
- Drop in total mortality when 3 percent of calories from processed meat are replaced with plant protein: 50 percent

STUDY 3: United States, 489,625 participants (Liao, 2019)

- Drop in colorectal cancer risk when red meat protein is replaced with plant protein: 11 percent*
- Drop in distal colon cancer risk when red meat protein is replaced with plant protein: 21 percent*
- Increase in distal colon cancer risk when plant protein is replaced with red meat: 23 percent**
- Drop in rectal cancer risk when red meat protein is replaced with plant protein: 16 percent*
- Increase in risk of rectal cancer when plant protein is replaced with red meat: 55 percent**

*Individuals in the highest versus lowest quintile (20 percent of group) of plant-protein intake.

**Individuals in the highest versus lowest quintile of animal protein intake.

STUDY 4: South Korea, meta-analysis of 43 studies, 16,572 participants (Kim, 2019)

- Drop in gastric cancer risk with every 3.5 ounces (100 g) per day of white meat consumed: 14 percent*
- Drop in gastric cancer risk in highest versus lowest categories of white-meat consumption: 20 percent*
- Increase in gastric cancer risk with every 3.5 ounces (100 g) per day of red meat consumed: 26 percent
- Increase in gastric cancer risk in highest versus lowest categories of red-meat consumption: 41 percent
- Increase in gastric cancer risk in highest versus lowest categories of processed-meat consumption: 57 percent
- Increase in gastric cancer risk with every 1.8 ounces (50 g) per day of processed meat consumed: 72 percent

*White meat, such as poultry and rabbit, may lower gastric cancer risk because it is lower in heme iron and saturated fat than red meat, and intake of white meat may indicate an overall healthier eating pattern.

STUDY 5: France, 61,476 participants (Diallo, 2018)

- Increase in overall cancer risk in the highest versus lowest quintile (20 percent of group) of red-meat intake: 31 percent
- Increase in breast cancer risk in the highest versus lowest quintile of red-meat intake: 79 percent

STUDY 6: China, Meta-analysis of 46 studies (Wu, 2016)

- Increase in breast cancer risk for every 1.8-ounce (50 g) serving of processed meat: 9 percent
- Increase in breast cancer risk for every 4-ounce (120 g) serving of red meat: 13 percent
- Drop in breast cancer risk for every serving (unspecified size) of soy food: 9 percent

STUDY 7: United States, 6,381 participants (Levine, 2014)

- Increase in cancer mortality in people aged 50–65 with medium protein intake (10–19 percent of calories from protein) compared to low intake (less than 10 percent of calories from protein): 306 percent (more than three times)
- Increase in cancer mortality in people aged 50–65 with high protein intake (more than 20 percent of calories from protein) compared to low intake (less than 10 percent of calories from protein): 433 percent (more than four times)

  Important caveat: Higher protein intakes were associated with increased risk of disease overall. However, that risk decreased or completely disappeared when the protein came from plants. In other words, the increased risk was with animal protein.

THE PLANT PROTEIN ADVANTAGE

The evidence favoring plant protein over animal protein for reducing disease risk extends beyond cardiovascular disease, type 2 diabetes, and cancer. The science suggests improved kidney function and a reduced risk of kidney stones, gallbladder disease, gout, inflammatory bowel diseases, and rheumatoid arthritis. Plant protein has the advantage over animal protein for two main reasons:

1. Plant foods are loaded with protective components that reduce the risk of chronic disease.
2. Plant foods contain few dietary components that increase the risk of chronic disease.

Diets high in animal products and refined carbohydrates lean in the opposite direction. They have few of the protective components that reduce disease risk and contain more potentially harmful components that increase disease risk. Table 6.1, below, summarizes the health effects of protective components and examines their relative content in plant foods and animal products. Table 6.2 on page 60 summarizes the health effects of potentially harmful dietary components and examines their relative content in plant foods and animal products.

TABLE 6.1. Health effects of protective components: Plant protein versus animal protein

FOOD COMPONENT	HEALTH EFFECTS	CONTENT IN PLANT PROTEIN*	CONTENT IN ANIMAL PROTEIN**
PROTECTIVE			
Antioxidants	Protect against free radicals and oxidative stress	Moderate to high	Low
Essential fatty acids	Protect against cardio-metabolic disorders, eye diseases, inflammatory diseases, and cognitive decline	High in seeds and walnuts; moderate in other plant foods	High in fish; variable in other animal products
Fiber	Improves the health of the gut microbiome, prevents gastrointestinal disorders, and reduces the risk of cancer, gallstones, cardiovascular disease, type 2 diabetes, and becoming overweight	High in legumes; moderate in nuts and seeds	Zero
Phytochemicals	Antioxidant, anti-inflammatory, anti-tumor, anticarcinogenic, antiviral, and antifungal	Moderate to high	Zero
Plant enzymes	Help convert phytochemicals into active forms; may aid digestion	Variable; notable sources include cruciferous and allium vegetables	Zero
Plant sterols	Reduce cholesterol absorption, blunt inflammation pathways, and support immune cell function	Moderate to high	Zero
Prebiotics	Support a healthy gut microbiome and provide food for friendly gut flora	High in legumes; moderate in nuts and seeds	Zero
Probiotics	Support a healthy gut microbiome	Variable; highest in fermented and cultured products	Variable; highest in fermented and cultured products

*Plant protein includes legumes (beans, dried peas, lentils, peanuts), nuts, and seeds.

**Animal protein includes meat (red and processed meat, and poultry), eggs, fish, and dairy products.

TABLE 6.2. Health effects of potentially harmful components: Plant protein versus animal protein

FOOD COMPONENT	HEALTH EFFECTS	CONTENT IN PLANT PROTEIN*	CONTENT IN ANIMAL PROTEIN**
POTENTIALLY HARMFUL			
Cholesterol	Modest adverse impact on blood cholesterol levels	Zero	Moderate in meat, poultry, fish and dairy, high in eggs
Endotoxins	Increase inflammation and disease risk	Low	Variable; highest in ground or processed meat products
Heme iron	Increases oxidative stress and the risk of related chronic diseases	Close to zero***	Moderate to high in meat, poultry and fish, little to none in eggs and dairy
Chemical contaminants	Increase oxidative stress and inflammation; disrupt hormones, damage vital organs, and damage DNA	Low to moderate	Moderate to high
Neu5Gc	Triggers inflammation and associated diseases	Zero	High in red meat; very low in poultry, fish, and eggs
Products of high temperature cooking (such as heterocyclic amines, polycyclic aromatic hydrocarbons, and advanced glycation end-products)	Promote oxidative stress and inflammation; increase risk of certain cancers, type 2 diabetes, Alzheimer's disease, and other chronic conditions	Generally low; varies with cooking methods; highest in fried or blackened foods; no heterocyclic amines	Generally moderate to high; varies with cooking methods; highest in processed, fried, or grilled meats
Saturated fat	Increases total and LDL cholesterol; reduces insulin sensitivity	Low	Moderate to high, except very low- or no-fat products such as certain fish and skim or 1% dairy
TMAO and precursors	Induce inflammation; contribute to plaque formation and kidney disease	Zero to very low	Low to high; TMAO is highest in fish; precursors are highest in red meat

*Plant protein sources include legumes (beans, dried peas, lentils, peanuts), nuts, and seeds.

**Animal protein sources include meat (red and processed meat, and poultry), eggs, fish, and dairy products.

***The Impossible Beef burger by Impossible Foods contains a relative of heme iron called leghemoglobin, found in the roots of legumes. Leghemoglobin has not been associated with adverse health effects.

CHOOSING PROTEIN FOR PROTECTION

The most protective sources of plant protein are those that give you the best bang for your buck, or the greatest health benefits per calorie. This means choosing protein-rich foods that are packed with fiber, antioxidants, phytochemicals, plant enzymes, plant sterols, pre- or probiotics, and micronutrients.

At the top of the list are legumes, such as beans, lentils, chickpeas, and split peas. These are linked with increased longevity and reduced disease risk. Next are minimally processed choices, such as traditional soy products like tofu and tempeh. These have a tremendous history of use among long-lived populations. Tempeh, a fermented product, is relatively high in fiber. Tofu is extremely versatile, provides readily available plant protein, and is lower in fiber. (For more on soy, see pages 26–28.)

Other lightly processed plant foods, such as hummus, seitan, and bean pasta, add variety and appeal to the diet. Hummus is popular, widely available in many flavors and variations, and easy to prepare at home. Commercial varieties can be high in sodium, so read the labels. Seitan is wheat protein and is a good source of leucine. You can make it at home or purchase it ready-made. Legume pastas, such as bean, lentil, or pea, are protein-rich replacements for traditional grain-based pastas. Bean pastas provide about half the carbohydrate, double the fiber, and triple the protein of regular pasta.

Veggie meats are concentrated sources of plant protein. They have a very low glycemic index (impact on blood glucose). However, they are more highly processed products, and some are low in fiber, and high in fat and sodium. Read the labels. In some products, the protein used has been extracted with harsh chemicals. To eliminate this concern, select organic products. Some veggie meats are whole-food based (such as burgers made with black beans and quinoa); these are great options. You also can assemble your own homemade versions.

Seeds and nuts deserve our attention. These provide significant amounts of protein and are important sources of healthy fats. For a ¼-cup (60 ml) serving, seeds have 8–13 grams of protein, and nuts 5–8 grams. The most protein-packed seeds are hemp and pumpkin seeds. The highest-protein nuts are almonds, black walnuts, and pistachios. Among the most healthful choices are seeds and nuts from the shell that are raw, soaked, dehydrated, or lightly roasted. Seed and nut butters without added fat and sugar are also great options. Minimize those that are flavored with salt, sugar, and chocolate. Seeds and nuts are high in calories, averaging between 175 and 200 calories in a ¼-cup (60 ml) serving, which is a moderate daily intake for people who are trying to shed excess weight.

References for this chapter are online at https://plant-poweredprotein.com/references.

7

Global Protein:
A Planet in Peril

The view of meat eating as a symbol of masculinity, status, and strength is deeply embedded into our culture. Yet, as the global population rises, this view becomes problematic because it's at odds with health, humanity, and the sustainability of fragile ecosystems. Over the past half century, the per capita protein supply has increased from both animal and plant sources. In most countries, increases in animal protein supply have outstripped those of plant protein.

In 1961, the average citizen of planet Earth had access to foods providing approximately 62 grams of protein per day. By 2013, that figure had risen to about 81 grams, an increase of about 32 percent. The supply of animal protein grew from about 0.7 ounce (20 g) per person per day in 1961 to approximately 1.1 ounces (32 g) in 2013, an increase of 63 percent. The supply of plant protein also rose from about 1.5 ounces (42 g) per person per day in 1961 to approximately 1.7 ounces (49 g) in 2013, an increase of 17 percent. Table 7.1 (page 63) provides comparisons between select countries. Note that the figures for individual countries are based on 2017 data, while world averages are based on 2013 data.

TABLE 7.1. Daily protein supply in grams in select countries*

COUNTRY	TOTAL PROTEIN 1961	TOTAL PROTEIN 2017	ANIMAL PROTEIN 1961	ANIMAL PROTEIN 2017	PLANT PROTEIN 1961	PLANT PROTEIN 2017
Australia	104.89	108.13	48.67	64.88	36.94	36.80
Brazil	56.24	90.86	17.79	52.80	38.45	38.06
Cambodia	41.72	65.40	3.99	19.61	37.73	46.24
Canada	91.13	101.20	58.32	50.97	32.82	50.23
China	39.00	101.35	3.20	40.44	35.80	60.92
Colombia	49.48	72.36	21.98	37.18	27.50	35.18
Denmark	82.33	113.05	47.20	73.23	35.12	39.81
Egypt	57.27	96.33	8.22	24.08	49.05	72.25
France	103.00	112.09	57.35	69.68	45.65	42.21
Germany	79.25	104.20	44.68	63.08	34.57	41.13
Ghana	41.54	62.96	12.33	15.35	29.21	47.61
Guatemala	51.31	69.88	11.08	21.53	40.23	48.35
Hong Kong	66.33	137.93	27.21	101.11	39.21	36.82
India	52.07	65.33	6.10	14.71	45.97	50.62
Iraq	48.68	60.55	13.81	13.55	34.87	47.00
Italy	82.54	106.75	29.03	57.04	53.51	49.71
Jamaica	51.91	72.85	23.15	35.92	28.76	36.93
Japan	74.19	86.58	24.56	48.07	49.63	38.51
Kenya	69.70	60.88	16.27	15.39	53.43	45.49
Mexico	62.62	93.40	16.16	43.79	46.45	49.61
Nepal	45.54	73.70	7.88	12.66	37.67	61.04
Philippines	41.42	62.68	15.32	25.71	26.11	36.97
Portugal	69.91	114.49	27.43	72.72	42.48	41.77
Samoa	45.00	85.75	21.50	51.01	23.51	32.74
South Korea	56.84	97.02	5.80	49.15	51.04	47.87
Spain	78.93	107.11	26.24	66.53	52.68	40.57
Thailand	42.30	61.00	11.44	26.18	30.86	34.82
Turkey	93.18	101.23	25.87	35.77	67.31	65.46
United States	95.21	113.73	62.99	73.87	32.22	39.86
Vietnam	45.47	90.03	8.89	36.81	36.58	53.22
Zambia	61.70	59.09	11.02	11.69	50.68	47.40
WORLD	61.46	81.23**	19.66	32.13**	41.80	49.10**

*A more comprehensive list is available at ourworldindata.org/food-supply.

**2017 figures are not available, so the 2013 figures were used in these cases.

Source: ourworldindata.org/food-supply.

If you examine this data, you will notice some interesting trends:

- China had the greatest increase in both total and animal protein supply. Total protein increased from 39 grams per person per day in 1961 to 101.35 grams in 2017—an increase of 160 percent. Animal protein supply jumped from 3.2 grams per person per day (the amount in less than ½ ounce of meat or poultry) to 40.44 grams per day. This is an increase of 1,164 percent. There was a more moderate increase in plant protein supply. Plant protein rose from 35.8 grams per person per day to 60.92 grams per day—a 70 percent jump.

- Many other Asian countries experienced a similar shift, though less extreme. In Cambodia, Thailand, and Vietnam, the increase in total protein supply ranged from 57 to 108 percent. Once again, the changes were greater for animal protein than for plant protein. The increases in animal protein supply ranged from 129 to 380 percent, while the increase in supply of plant protein ranged from 13 to 45 percent.

- The relative supply of animal to plant protein is generally lower in Asian and African countries than in wealthier countries. Often, the plant protein supply is two or three times greater than the animal protein supply. Hong Kong is a notable exception with more than 100 grams of animal protein per person per day, and 37 grams of plant protein per day.

In wealthier regions, such as North America, Europe, and Australia, animal protein accounted for about two-thirds of the total protein consumed. Canada is an exception, with animal and plant protein contributing equally to total protein intake.

- The supply of both animal and plant protein has increased in many but not all developing countries. For example, in Samoa, total protein increased from 45 to almost 86 grams per person per day. Animal protein increased from 22 to 51 grams per person per day, and plant protein increased from 23 to 34 grams per person per day. By contrast, in Zambia, changes in protein supply were minimal. Total protein per person per day decreased by about 2 grams. Animal protein increased by less than a gram and plant protein decreased by about 3 grams.

- As per capita income increases, the demand for meat rises, yet there are significant differences in local dietary preferences. Populations that have long relied on legumes as dietary staples continue to eat more plant than animal protein or to consume similar quantities of each.

DISCUSSION

If our current trajectory remains unchanged, the health and ecological impacts of our protein choices will be grim. In response, key organizations are taking action to curb the appetite for animal protein. Some of the most notable are featured below:

INTERNATIONAL REPORTS

EAT-Lancet Commission on Food, Planet, Health (2019)

The EAT-Lancet Commission on Food, Planet, Health brought together 37 multiple-disciplinary, multicultural scientists from 16 countries to answer one question: Can we feed a future population of 10 billion people a healthy diet within planetary boundaries? The report summarizes the challenges we face:

> Food is the single strongest lever to optimize human health and environmental sustainability on Earth. However, food is currently threatening both people and the planet. An immense challenge facing humanity is to provide a growing world population with healthy diets from sustainable food systems. While global food production of calories has generally kept pace with population growth, more than 820 million people still lack sufficient food, and many more consume either low-quality diets or too much food. Unhealthy diets now pose a greater risk to morbidity and mortality than unsafe sex, alcohol, drug, and tobacco use combined. Global food production threatens climate stability and ecosystem resilience and constitutes the single largest driver of environmental degradation and transgression of planetary boundaries. Taken together the outcome is dire. A radical transformation of the global food system is urgently needed. Without action, the world risks failing to meet the UN Sustainable Development Goals (SDGs) and the Paris Agreement, and today's children will inherit a planet that has been severely degraded and where much of the population will increasingly suffer from malnutrition and preventable disease.

The commission recommends a shift toward a diet rich in plant-based foods with fewer animal-sourced foods. This type of diet provides notable benefits for human and planetary health. To achieve this, the commission suggests doubling our intake of healthy foods, such as fruits, vegetables, legumes, and nuts. It urges cutting less healthful foods, such as red meat and added sugars, by 50 percent.

World Health Organization/FAO, Sustainable Healthy Diets: Guiding Principles (2019)

This joint WHO/FAO report provides guiding principles for sustainable, healthy dietary patterns. It takes all dimensions of individuals' health and well-being into consideration. The most impressive diets have low environmental pressure and impact. They are accessible, affordable, safe, equitable, and culturally acceptable.

As populations become more affluent and urbanized, they demand more food, particularly more meat, fish, dairy, eggs, sugar, fats, and oils. This dietary transition is associated with increased risk of diet-related diseases, while the animal-sourced foods have higher environmental impacts per calorie or grams of food produced than do most plant-based foods. In addition, projected population growth of two billion people by 2050, most of which is likely to occur in currently low and middle-income countries, will further increase diet-related environmental pressure. . . . Many studies have shown that reducing meat consumption can reduce GHGs while remaining nutritionally adequate. For example, global adoption of a low-meat diet that meets nutritional recommendations for fruits, vegetables, and caloric requirements is estimated to reduce diet-related GHGs by nearly 50 percent, and premature mortality by nearly 20 percent.

IPCC Special Report: Climate Change and Land (2019)

The Intergovernmental Panel on Climate Change (IPCC) put out a special report in 2019 that declared the answer to the climate change crisis is on our plates. According to this report, the food supply is responsible for 21–37 percent of global GHG emissions. It suggests that a shift toward plant-based diets is one of the most significant ways to reduce GHGs from the agriculture sector. The report describes a healthy, sustainable diet as high in coarse grains, pulses (legumes), fruits and vegetables, and nuts and seeds, and low in energy-intensive, animal-sourced foods and discretionary items, such as sugary beverages.

Food and Agriculture Organization of the United Nations (FAO), the Food Climate Research Network—Plates, Pyramids, Planet (2016)

In this joint publication, forward-thinking governments that integrate nutrition science with sustainable food systems are highlighted. The official dietary guidelines of Germany, Brazil, Sweden, and Qatar all promote plant-rich diets:

- **Germany:** Choose mainly plant-based foods. They have a health-promoting effect and foster a sustainable diet.
- **Brazil:** Base diets on many varieties of natural or minimally processed foods mainly of plant origin. Reduced consumption and therefore production of animal foods will reduce emissions of the greenhouse gases responsible for global warming.
- **Sweden:** Eat less meat; choose plant food instead. Try to exchange one or two meals of beef, lamb, pork, or chicken every week with vegetarian meals, or eat smaller portions of meat.

- **Qatar:** Emphasize a plant-based diet, including vegetables, fruit, whole-grain cereals, legumes, nuts, and seeds. Reduce leftovers and waste.

This document emphasizes the need for populations to shift to more sustainable diets and food systems. The report points out that dietary patterns with low environmental impacts are also good for health. It says diets that achieve a win on all fronts are based on plant foods, including minimally processed tubers and whole grains, legumes, fruits, vegetables, and unsalted seeds and nuts.

NATIONAL EFFORTS (Not Highlighted in Plates, Pyramids, Planet)

Health Canada, Canada's Dietary Guidelines and Canada's Food Guide (2019)

Canada's latest dietary guidelines and food guide issued in 2019 are focused on healthy eating and optimizing health outcomes. Environmental sustainability considerations are also woven in. The foundation for healthy eating includes a series of guidelines, with the first being: Nutritious foods are the foundation for healthy eating. Here is what the guidelines also say.

- Vegetables, fruit, whole grains, and protein foods should be consumed regularly. Among protein foods, consume plant-based foods more often.
- Protein foods include legumes, nuts, seeds, tofu, fortified soy beverages, fish, shellfish, eggs, poultry, lean red meat including wild game, lower-fat milk, lower-fat yogurts, lower-fat kefir, and cheeses lower in fat and sodium.
- Foods that contain mostly unsaturated fat should replace foods that contain mostly saturated fat.
- Water should be the beverage of choice.

Health Canada, the national health department, also provides environmental impact considerations. The document states: "There are potential environmental benefits to improving current patterns of eating as outlined in this report. For example, there is evidence supporting a lesser environmental impact of patterns of eating higher in plant-based foods and lower in animal-based foods. The potential benefits include helping to conserve soil, water, and air."

Swiss Food Pyramid (2016)

The Swiss Food Pyramid provides recommendations for a healthy and enjoyable diet. It suggests a range of intake for various food groups. Unsweetened beverages (preferably water), daily physical activity, and sufficient relaxation are recommended. The guide discusses the impacts of our food choices on the environment.

It advocates sustainable eating, including avoiding food waste, a preference for plant-based foods, and foods that are environment and animal friendly, seasonal, regional, and in compliance with fair-trade principles.

China's Dietary Guidelines (2016)

As with other national guidelines, the emphasis of this document is on improving the health of the population. It suggests the entire population reduce meat intake by 50 percent by 2030. If China succeeds in this quest, it would be a monumental contribution to curbing climate change, as well as its looming health crisis.

It may come as a surprise to learn that in absolute terms, China is the world's largest consumer of meat. Their rapidly rising living standards have meant more meat, despite a long history of plant-based eating. With education campaigns, plant-based alternatives are piquing the interest of health-conscious consumers.

WE HAVE A CHOICE!

When we consider the consequences of our food choices, for ourselves, and beyond ourselves, eating plants makes sense. Every person who shifts in this direction is helping to sustain a growing population on a shrinking planet. We are standing at a crossroads. By choosing plant protein, we are giving future generations a fighting chance.

References for this chapter are online at https://plant-poweredprotein.com/references.

Protein during Pregnancy and Lactation

Natalya was thrilled to learn that she was pregnant after almost two years of trying. She and her husband, Chris, had been 100 percent plant-based for about a year and a half and they had their hearts set on raising children this way. The plant-based kids within their circle of friends seemed perfectly happy and healthy. So, when they discussed their dietary choice with their obstetrician, they were taken aback by her concern. She encouraged Natalya to add fish and eggs back into her diet to ensure sufficient protein and essential amino acids. Natalya and Chris decided to embark on a mission to get as much information as possible. They were determined to effectively address the obstetrician's concerns at their next visit. Natalya told Chris that if after their research she was not sufficiently reassured, she would include small amounts of animal products during her pregnancy. Natalya vowed not to do anything that could potentially harm their baby.

Protein had not worried Natalya and Chris. In the plant-based world, the mantra seemed to be that if you get enough calories, you get enough protein. They gathered several trusted resources and were surprised to learn how critical protein is during stages of rapid growth and development. Extra protein provides building blocks for the baby's skeleton, skin, muscles, and other budding body parts. It is required for the mother's expanding uterus, breast tissue, blood volume, and body fluids. About 40 percent of this increased protein will be used for the baby, and the remaining 60 percent will be used for the mother.

Natalya and Chris were curious to know exactly how much extra protein would be needed to ensure a healthy pregnancy. They turned to the recommended dietary allowances (RDA) for this information. They learned that the RDA for expectant mothers is close to 50 percent higher than it is for nonpregnant women. This makes perfect sense when you consider the amount of growth that occurs in both mother and baby. The protein RDA (based on healthy pre-pregnancy weight) is 0.5 grams per pound of body weight per day (1.1 g per kg) during pregnancy and 0.59 grams per pound of body weight per day (1.3 g per kg) during lactation. This compares to 0.36 grams per pound per day (0.8 g per kg) for nonpregnant, nonlactating women. Natalya and Chris discovered that the digestibility of protein is slightly lower from whole plant foods than from animal products. This is due to the fiber present in plants. For people eating plant-based diets, adding 10 percent to the recommended dietary allowance compensates for this. This translates to about 0.5 grams per pound (1.2 g per kg) of protein daily of pre-pregnancy body weight. This addition may not be necessary for people who eat several servings each day of low-fiber, high-protein plant foods, such as tofu, soy milk, veggie meats, and plant-protein powders. Nor does it apply to lacto-ovo vegetarians or pescatarians, who consume some animal products. However, adding 10 percent to the recommended dietary allowance is a safe and reasonable choice for all plant-based eaters. To calculate your personal protein needs, see figure 6.1, below.

FIGURE 6.1. Calculating your recommended protein intake on a plant-based diet.

EXAMPLE: For Natalya, or a plant-based woman whose pre-pregnancy weight is 125 pounds (57 kg*):

Multiply 57 kg x 1.2 g/kg = 68 g

FOR YOURSELF: Multiply your pre-pregnancy weight by 1.2 g/kg to get your recommended protein intake for the day:

Your weight in kg _____ x 1.2 g/kg/day = _____

*1 kg = 2.2 pounds; your weight in pounds (lb.) ÷ 2.2 = weight in kilograms (kg)

Another way of calculating your approximate protein requirement is to add 25 grams per day to the nonpregnant protein requirement, or 50 grams for women who are expecting twins. This provides a slightly different but still acceptable number. Women eating 100 percent plant-based diets can increase these figures by 10 percent.

Table 8.1, below, summarizes the recommendations for protein intakes during pregnancy and lactation. Table 8.2 on page 71 provides recommended intakes for women of different healthy body weights.

TABLE 8.1. Protein needs during pregnancy and lactation

	NONPREGNANT WOMEN	PREGNANT WOMEN	LACTATING WOMEN
RDA (g/kg/day)	0.8	1.1	1.3
RDA + 10% (for plant-based) g/kg/day	0.9	1.2	1.4

TABLE 8.2. Pregnancy protein RDA at different healthy body weights

HEALTHY BODY WEIGHT*	RECOMMENDED PROTEIN INTAKE (healthy body weight x 1.1 g/kg*)	RECOMMENDED PLANT-BASED PROTEIN INTAKE (healthy body weight x 1.2 g/kg*)
50 kg (110 lb.)	55	60
55 kg (121 lb.)	60.5	66
60 kg (132 lb.)	66	72
65 kg (143 lb.)	71.5	78
70 kg (154 lb.)	77	84
75 kg (165 lb.)	82.5	90
80 kg (176 lb.)	88	96
85 kg (187 lb.)	93.5	102

*A healthy body weight for most women will fall into a healthy body mass index (BMI) range. You can estimate your range by using a BMI calculator online. For example, if you are five feet, four inches tall, a healthy BMI for you would be between 108 and 145 pounds. Generally, healthy body weight will lean toward the lower end of this range for small-framed women and the upper end of this range for large-framed women.

After learning about her protein requirements, Natalya wondered about some of the larger women in her prenatal class. Her friend Sarah's pre-pregnancy weight was 176 pounds (80 kg) and her pre-pregnancy BMI was 28.6, which is in the "overweight" zone. Should Sarah base her protein RDA on her pre-pregnancy weight? This is where things get a little tricky. The body weight used in the calculations for the protein RDA is "healthy body weight." Of course, there is a range of healthy body weights for individuals of different heights and frame sizes. So, determining a person's healthy body weight is subjective. Generally, a person can select a weight that they feel is the healthiest for them—it should fall somewhere in the healthy BMI range of 18.6–24.9. Sarah feels her healthiest weight is 145 pounds (66 kg), so she would use the 66 kilogram figure for her calculations. Her RDA based on 1.1 grams per kilogram of body weight would be 73 grams. Sarah would not add 10 percent to her calculations, as she eats an omnivorous diet.

Natalya and Chris also wondered if plant foods provide enough essential amino acids. They discovered that needs for specific essential amino acids do rise in both pregnancy and lactation. However, built into the RDA is the assumption that the increase in protein intake will ensure ample essential amino acids. In plant-based diets, it is helpful to include sufficient foods from the legume family, such as beans, lentils, split peas, tofu, tempeh, and peanuts.

The bottom line is that Natalya will need to consume more protein-rich foods during both pregnancy and lactation, as should nonvegetarian women. How can she achieve the recommended protein intakes? During pregnancy and lactation, it is important to include excellent sources of protein at each meal and in most snacks. For practical guidelines, see our top 10 tips for boosting plant protein on pages 105–107. For sample menus providing 60, 80, and 100 grams of protein per day, see pages 108–109. With a little planning, it is easy to get enough protein from plant foods—even without protein powders.

SHOULD PROTEIN POWDERS BE USED TO BOOST PROTEIN DURING PREGNANCY AND LACTATION?

The most healthful way to increase protein intake is to be generous with high-protein plant foods, such as tofu, lentils, beans, and hemp seeds. Veggie meat substitutes can add a further boost, if desired. Protein supplements are generally unnecessary, though they can be helpful for some people. Whole plant foods provide fiber, phytochemicals, and antioxidants, and they are rich sources of vitamins and minerals. Many protein powders contain added sugars, colors, artificial flavors, thickeners, herbs, caffeine, and artificial sweeteners. Vitamin and mineral fortification can boost intakes beyond the upper limits, especially when prenatal supplements are factored in. In addition, protein powders, including organic products, may contain contaminants, such as heavy metals, bisphenol A (BPA), and pesticides. If you or your health-care provider feel a supplement is warranted, do some digging before purchasing. Select a product that contains a mix of plant proteins, is free of unnecessary additions, and contains low levels of contaminants. Looking at a label won't tell you whether a product contains these contaminants. Look for a third-party certification stamp on the label to ensure the product has been screened for safety.

In the end, Natalya and Chris were grateful for the nudge from the obstetrician. The protein investigation heightened their awareness of its importance during stages of growth. Natalya and Chris developed a greater appreciation for legumes, including soy foods such as tofu, edamame, and soy milk. Natalya was completely reassured that plant foods could provide enough protein and essential amino acids.

As a bonus, they discovered several potential advantages of plant-based pregnancies. Mothers who consume 100 percent plant-based diets have fewer caesarean deliveries, less postpartum depression, and lower rates of neonatal and maternal mortality. Plant-based diets protect against preeclampsia, pre-pregnancy obesity, and exposure to chemicals that can damage DNA. One study reported that the highest value for six contaminants in the breast milk of vegans was lower than the lowest value from the breast milk of omnivores. She was more convinced than ever that her dietary choices would protect the precious little person she was carrying.

References for this chapter are online at https://plant-poweredprotein.com/references.

Infants and Toddlers: (Birth to Age 3)

Brittany and Priya were two remarkable moms. When Aaron arrived, they were instantly smitten. Brittany gave birth to the baby but both moms shared in breastfeeding. Yes, it is possible! Brittany's and Priya's diets were completely plant based. They wanted to make sure Aaron would get everything he needed to grow healthy and strong without using animal products. They wondered if plant protein would provide all the essential amino acids little ones need. They planned to breastfeed for at least two years, but they didn't know which plant-based milks would be best to offer him in addition during the toddler years. They wondered if they could use soy formula to supplement breast milk if necessary. They had read on several websites that soy might not be safe. Some websites talked about possible feminizing effects. Brittany and Priya decided to see a plant-based registered dietitian to help them answer these questions.

Infancy is the stage of life when growth is the fastest. Adults need 11–18 calories per pound (25–40 calories per kg) of body weight, while newborns require more than 45 calories per pound (100 calories per kg). Toddlers aged one to three years need about 38 calories per pound (83 calories per kg). Protein provides the building blocks for that growth, so adequate protein at this stage of life is critical.

HOW MUCH PROTEIN DO INFANTS AND TODDLERS REQUIRE?

Birth to Six Months

During this stage, an adequate intake (AI) is used rather than a recommended dietary allowance (RDA). The AI is a "best guess," based on the protein intake of healthy infants drinking only human milk, which is recommended—1.52 grams per kilogram of body weight per day. This means that a 10-pound (4.5 kg) baby needs about 7 grams of protein per day. Plant-based breastfeeding moms may wonder if their baby gets enough protein. It is reassuring to know that a mother's diet does affect her milk, but it does not affect the protein content. Commercial infant formula has 40–60 percent more protein than breast milk. Yet the difference in protein content does not adversely affect the baby's protein status. This is because the protein in breast milk is much more digestible.

Seven Months to One Year

From seven months to one year of age, babies ingest significant amounts of protein through solid foods. However, breast milk or infant formula continue to be vital staples until at least twelve months of age. From six to eight months, breast milk accounts for about 80 percent of a baby's calories, gradually declining to about 50 percent by one year. At the stage of seven months to one year, the recommended dietary allowance is 1.2 grams of protein per kilogram body weight or 11 grams of protein per day for an infant who weighs 20 pounds (9 kg). Most infants exceed recommended intakes, with about 7 grams of protein coming from milk or formula and another 7 grams or more from solid foods.

One to Three Years

In toddlers aged one to three years, growth is slower than in the first year of life. During this stage, the recommended dietary allowance of protein is 1.05 grams per kilogram of body weight per day. A boy or girl who weighs 27 pounds (12.3 kg) needs about 13 grams of protein per day. For children who eat mostly or exclusively plant foods, some experts recommend adding 30 percent to the recommended dietary allowance. This is because of the reduced digestibility of protein from plants. This may be more than is required for toddlers who receive breast milk or formula daily. It also may be more than is needed for lacto-ovo vegetarian toddlers, and for toddlers who regularly eat high-protein, low-fiber plant foods, such as tofu, soy milk, and veggie meats. An increase of 15–20 percent may be enough for these children. Adding 30 percent to the recommended dietary allowance means 1.36 grams per kilogram of body weight per day or 17 grams of protein per day for a 27-pound (12.3 kg) child. A 15–20 percent increase would mean a total of 15 grams per day.

PROTEIN INTAKES OF PLANT-BASED TODDLERS VERSUS OMNIVOROUS TODDLERS

The VeChi Youth Study from Germany is the largest study to compare protein intakes of toddlers aged one to three years. It included 139 vegan, 127 lacto-ovo vegetarian, and 164 nonvegetarian children. The children in all three groups grew normally. At this age, the recommended dietary allowance for protein is 1.05 grams per kilogram of body weight per day. On average, the toddlers consumed more than double the protein recommended dietary allowance, regardless of their dietary category. The study's authors concluded that vegetarian and vegan diets in early childhood provide about the same energy and macronutrients as nonvegetarian diets and support normal growth and development.

BRITTANY AND PRIYA'S VISIT WITH THE DIETITIAN

Brittany and Priya were excited to discover that an experienced plant-based dietitian, Martha Chen, had an office close by. Aaron was four months old and exclusively breastfeeding at the time of their consultation, so he was still a couple of months away from beginning solid foods. They asked Martha for assistance with menu planning and for answers to three burning questions. Martha's answers took a huge load off their shoulders.

Q: *Is it necessary to serve Aaron complementary proteins when he starts eating solid foods?*

A: Martha explained that protein complementation at each meal is not usually necessary. Brittany and Priya do need to ensure that Aaron gets a variety of plant foods and enough calories each day. Martha showed them the Plant-Based Plate (page 102). She went over the food groups and appropriate intakes from each group. She provided a few sample menus to assist them with meal planning (see chapter 13).

Martha explained that lysine is the essential amino acid that tends to fall short for children eating restrictive diets. For example, toddlers who are fed mainly rice with little else may not get quite enough lysine. She told them they could ensure sufficient lysine by including legumes with meals at least two or three times a day. Beans, lentils, and split peas are great choices. Legumes can take the form of soy milk, soy yogurt, tofu, tempeh, and veggie meats. Seeds and nuts, or their butters or cheeses, and pseudograins, such as quinoa, also can contribute significantly to intake. (See pages 24–25 for lysine content of common plant foods.) The recommended dietary allowance for lysine in toddlers one to three years old is 58 milligrams per gram of protein required. So, a toddler who weighs 27 pounds (12.3 kg) and needs 17 grams of protein per day would require an estimated 986 milligrams of lysine (58 x 17) each day. Consuming just ¼ cup (60 ml) of firm tofu (556 mg lysine), and ⅓ cup (85 ml) of cooked navy beans (460 mg lysine) would provide about 1,016 milligrams of lysine. Other plant foods would contribute to overall lysine intake as well. It is important to note that grains tend to have relatively low levels of lysine, so grain-heavy diets can more easily fall short. For example, a child would get just 153 milligrams of lysine from 1 cup (250 ml) of cooked white rice.

Q: *How old does Aaron need to be before consuming plant-based milks as his primary beverage, apart from water? What types of plant-based milks are most appropriate for babies and toddlers?*

A: Once a baby starts solid foods, plant milks can be used in food preparation. These milks must not replace formula or breast milk during the first year of life. For breastfed babies, continue breastfeeding during the toddler years, if possible. For formula-fed babies, formula can be stopped at one year or provided during the second year of life. This can help bridge nutritional gaps for days when food intake is poor. When fully plant-based babies wean from the breast or stop taking formula, full-fat fortified soy milk or pea milk are acceptable alternatives. These milks provide protein, calcium, vitamin D, and vitamin B_{12}. Other fortified nondairy milks, such as almond, cashew, oat, or coconut, do not provide adequate protein to serve as primary milks for toddlers. However, they are safe for occasional use in recipes. Table 9.1 (page 77) provides a nutritional comparison of various milks, both nondairy and dairy. Note that the nondairy milks used in this chart are all fortified. Unfortified milks are not recommended for toddlers (or older children), as they are low in calcium and do not have vitamin D or vitamin B_{12} added. The calcium content of fortified milks usually ranges from 300 to 465 milligrams per cup (250 ml), which is similar to or higher than cow's milk (check labels). Iron, which is a critical nutrient for infants and toddlers, is higher in most plant milks than in cow's milk (see table 9.1, page 77). The amount of added sugar in milks varies widely. Unsweetened milks have no added sugar and are generally good choices. "Original" milks have about the same amount of sugar as lactose in cow's milk. These are also good choices, especially for small children who need extra calories. One cup (250 ml) of original soy milk has five grams of sugar (just more than 1 t./5 ml). By comparison, 1 cup of soda has 28–32 grams of added sugar (7–8 t./35–40 ml)! Flavored milks, such as sweetened vanilla or chocolate, have higher amounts of added sugars. For example, vanilla almond milk typically contains about 16 grams, or about 4 teaspoons, of added sugar. These sweeter milks are not generally recommended. Be sure to read labels!

Q: *Will soy foods such as tofu and soy milk cause feminization or interfere with Aaron's development? Is soy formula safe for babies?*

A: Martha explained that soy does not cause feminization of males at usual intake levels. (See page 27 for further information.) Soy does not lower testosterone

TABLE 9.1. Comparing milks for nutrients per cup

MILK	CALORIES	PROTEIN (GRAMS)	FAT (GRAMS)	CALCIUM (MG)	VITAMIN A (MCG)	VITAMIN D (IU)	VITAMIN B$_{12}$ (MCG)	IRON (MG)
Whole cow's milk	149	8	8	276	46	128	1.1	0.07
Soy milk, original, fortified	110	8	4.5	450	150	120	3	1.3
Soy milk, unsweetened, fortified	80	7	4	300	150	120	3	1
Pea milk, original, fortified	90	8	4.5	465	110	240	2.5	0
Pea milk, unsweetened, fortified	70	8	4.5	465	110	240	2.5	0
Almond milk, original, fortified	60	1	2.5	450	150	100	0	0.5
Almond milk, unsweetened, fortified	30	1	2.5	450	150	100	0	0.5
Cashew milk, unsweetened	25	1	2	450	150	100	0	0.5
Oat milk, original	80	2	3	460	230	160	2.4	0.7
Oat milk, unsweetened	60	1	3	460	225	160	2.4	0.7
Coconut milk, original	70	0	4.5	460	180	80	0.9	0.6
Coconut milk, unsweetened	40	0	4	460	180	80	0.9	0.5

Sources: US Department of Agriculture, Agricultural Research Service. FoodData Central, 2019 (fdc.nal.usda.gov); nutrition facts from company websites (Silk brand for soy, almond, cashew, oat, and coconut; Ripple brand for pea milk).

levels, raise estrogen levels, or reduce sperm count. Nor does soy cause males to grow "man breasts." Soy foods are safe and nutritious as part of a varied, healthful diet (see pages 26–28 for more information on soy). In fact, soy consumption in childhood has been shown to reduce the risk of cancer in later life.

Brittany and Priya were also curious about the safety of soy formula, in case they needed to supplement their breastfeeding. Martha reassured them that the American Academy of Pediatrics considers soy formula safe for full-term infants. Human studies have found little or no difference in sexual development, thyroid function, brain development, or the immune systems in babies fed soy formula compared to those fed cow's milk–based formula. Although soy formula is higher in aluminum than breast milk or cow's milk formula, the amount is within safe limits for full-term infants. Soy formula is not recommended for preterm infants weighing less than 4 pounds (1,800 g), babies with compromised kidney function, or infants who have congenital hypothyroidism.

Brittany and Priya now felt confident that they could provide ample protein and essential amino acids for Aaron. They were excited to come up with creative ways of making legumes and legume-based products daily favorites for their little boy.

ENSURING SUFFICIENT PROTEIN DURING THE FIRST THREE YEARS

There are many ways that plant-based parents can ensure their little ones get plenty of protein. Begin by including protein with each meal and with some of the snacks. Since protein requirements for toddlers are small, the amounts add up quickly. Don't stress too much if intakes vary from day to day; this is normal. Instead, focus on providing a variety of nutritious foods. The Plant-Based Plate, our food guide on pages 101–103, will help you to do just that. Of course, the serving sizes are smaller for toddlers. Your little one will let you know when she or he has eaten enough. For practical ways of boosting protein, see our top 10 tips on pages 105–107. To calculate your toddler's protein intake, you might look up amounts in table 4.1 on pages 32–39.

References for this chapter are online at https://plant-poweredprotein.com/references.

10

Children and Teens: Ages 4–18

Amy and D'Andre had been married for five years. They had a beautiful, blended family with four children—16-year-old Trayvon, 14-year-old Aisha, 11-year-old Lucas, and 6-year-old Olivia. They began their transition to plant-based eating about two years after getting married. The shift was initiated by Trayvon, who was a soft-hearted, animal rights eco-warrior. Trayvon loved watching documentaries and it didn't take him long to make the connection between food, farm animals, and climate change. When he announced that he would no longer eat meat, Amy and D'Andre felt exasperated. Feeding a large family was enough of a challenge without having to buy and prepare separate food for one family member.

When Trayvon's thirteenth birthday approached, his parents asked him what he would like. Trayvon responded that his one wish was for them to watch his favorite documentary, *The Game Changers*. That one film rocked their world. They embarked on a mission to learn more, and soon found themselves gravitating to plant-based eating. Aisha and Lucas were resistant. Olivia, who was only three years old at the time, was unfazed. Amy and D'Andre decided that they would transition slowly, as the children were ready. For a while they purchased just enough animal products to appease their diehard meat and dairy eaters. As time went on, Aisha and Lucas became more open to eating meat alternatives and to learning more about plant-based living. One of the most powerful influences for Aisha was a trip to an animal sanctuary while they were on summer vacation. Aisha bonded with a pig named Wilbur and lost her lust for bacon and ham. In time, the whole family was on board.

Children and teens are the ultimate "bodybuilders." They are forming muscles and bones at remarkable rates. A 3-year-old child measuring 37 inches (94 cm) and weighing about 30 pounds (13.6 kg) will gain about 26 inches (66 cm) in height and 75 pounds (34 kg) in weight by 13 years of age. This takes some impressive building blocks, all of which are derived from food. Poor nutrition, including suboptimal protein intakes, can compromise growth and development. Fortunately, plant-based diets provide sufficient calories and variety to cover all the bases.

HOW MUCH PROTEIN DO CHILDREN AND TEENS REQUIRE?

When Amy and D'Andre began transitioning to plant-based eating, they were worried that their children might not get enough protein. They had believed the conventional wisdom that people need meat for protein and that getting enough protein from plants was tricky, especially for growing children. They wondered if vegetarians had to carefully combine foods to ensure sufficient protein. Amy and D'Andre were relieved to learn that plants could provide ample protein, even for children.

The recommended dietary allowance (RDA) for protein is 0.95 grams per kilogram of body weight per day for children aged 4–13 years, and 0.85 grams for teens 14–18 years of age. Some experts suggest adding 15–20 percent for plant-based children ages 4–18 years, and 30 percent for toddlers ages 1–3 years. This addition helps to compensate for the reduced digestibility of protein from fiber-rich plants. For children who regularly include animal products, such as milk and eggs, no increase is required. For children who eat generous amounts of lower-fiber plant foods, such as soy or pea milk, tofu, veggie meats, seitan, and peanut butter, smaller increases of about 10 percent may be sufficient. However, for children who eat mainly unprocessed plant foods, these increases are reasonable and achievable. Recommended protein intakes, including those suggested for 100 percent plant-based eaters, are summarized in table 10.1 (page 81).

HOW PROTEIN INTAKES OF PLANT-BASED YOUTH COMPARE TO THOSE OF OMNIVOROUS YOUTH

The most robust study comparing nutrient intakes of children and teens eating plant-based and omnivorous diets is the VeChi Youth Study from 2021. This study examined dietary intakes of 401 German children from 6 to 18 years of age, including 115 vegans, 149 lacto-ovo vegetarians, and 137 omnivores. Protein intakes were 1.16 grams per kilogram of body weight for vegans, 1.14 grams for lacto-ovo vegetarians, and 1.36 grams for omnivores. If we add 20 percent to the protein recommended dietary allowance for 4-to-8-year-old children, it would rise from 0.95 grams to 1.14 grams. If we add 15 percent to the protein recommended dietary allowance for 9-to-13-year-old children, it would rise from 0.95 grams to 1.09 grams. For teens, the recommended dietary allowance may be increased by 15 percent from 0.85 grams to 0.98 grams. The average intakes in the VeChi study all exceeded these adjusted plant-exclusive recommendations. However, the adjusted recommendation (1.14 g/kg/day) for children aged 4–8 is just slightly below the average intakes in the VeChi study of 1.16 grams. This suggests that parents

TABLE 10.1. Recommended protein intakes for typical weights during childhood and adolescence

AGE, YEARS	PROTEIN RDA G/KG/DAY	BODY WEIGHT KILOGRAMS (POUNDS)	PROTEIN RDA GRAMS/DAY	SUGGESTED % INCREASE FOR 100% PLANT-BASED	RECOMMENDED FOR 100% PLANT-BASED GRAMS/DAY
4–8	0.95	15 (33)	14	20%	17
		20 (44)	19		23
		25 (55)	24		29
9–13	0.95	30 (66)	29	15%	33
		35 (77)	33		38
		40 (88)	38		44
		45 (99)	43		49
14–18	0.85	50 (110)	43	15%	49
		55 (121)	47		54
		60 (132)	51		59
		65 (143)	55		63
		70 (154)	60		69
		75 (165)	64		74

do need to be conscious of including sufficient protein, particularly for younger children. It is reassuring that vegan youth (6–18 years) had the highest intakes of vitamin A, thiamin, folate, vitamin C, vitamin E, magnesium, iron, and zinc. They also had the highest intakes of fiber, and the lowest intakes of added sugars (almost half that of others), and total and saturated fat. Youth in all dietary groups had low intakes of vitamin D and riboflavin, although dietary intakes were lowest among the vegans. Vegans also had low dietary intakes of B_{12} and calcium. However, lab measures did not show deficiencies in vitamin B_{12} as supplements were typically used.

THE LONG-TERM HEALTH CONSEQUENCES OF SWAPPING OUT ANIMAL FOR PLANT PROTEIN

Amy and D'Andre wondered if removing animal protein could negatively impact the health of their children in the long term. They asked their plant-based family doctor, who explained that the long-term health consequences of getting protein from plants are favorable. Plant eaters experience a lower risk of chronic diseases and becoming overweight. Plant-based children may experience a slightly delayed onset of puberty, while children eating the greatest amounts of animal products experience earlier puberty. Early onset of puberty is associated with an increased risk of hormone-related cancers, metabolic syndrome, cardiovascular disease, and all causes of mortality. Clearly, protein-rich plant foods provide protection over the long term.

UNIQUE CHALLENGES

Each of Amy and D'Andre's children had unique protein challenges. Trayvon, who wanted to add muscle to his thin frame, wondered if protein powders might help. Aisha was conscious about fitting in with friends and did not want to appear different from her peers. Lucas was a picky eater and had never been a fan of beans. Olivia had an allergy to cashews. Amy and D'Andre did what they could to be supportive in each of these situations. Let's explore the strategies they used in each case.

Trayvon: Muscle-Making Mission

Trayvon was both compassionate and competitive. He was an exceptional soccer player and was on an elite rep team. Trayvon was fit but he wanted to build more muscle for power and speed. One of his buddies suggested that his vegan diet may have been the reason why he wasn't muscular. Trayvon hoped to prove that he could gain muscle without eating meat. When Trayvon asked his parents if they would buy him protein powder, they suggested getting some expert advice. He agreed and they booked consultations with Alejandro Sanchez, a dietitian and sports nutrition specialist. Alejandro suggested that Trayvon aim for 1.5 grams of protein per kilogram of body weight. Trayvon was 5 feet, 10 inches tall and weighed 143 pounds (65 kg). This meant he needed to eat at least 98 grams of protein per day. Trayvon was currently eating about 75 grams of protein per day. Alejandro worked with Trayvon to develop menus that would help him reach his protein target. Some of the protein-boosting strategies suggested are outlined below. While Trayvon could choose to do all of them, selecting just two or three per day would be enough to reach his daily target of 98 grams of protein:

1. **Add protein to breakfast.** Trayvon's standard breakfast was a bowl of cereal with a sliced banana and almond milk, and two pieces of toast with margarine and jam. Switching to soy milk, adding 2 tablespoons (30 ml) hemp seeds to his cereal, and swapping the margarine for 2 tablespoons (30 ml) peanut butter added 21 grams of protein to breakfast.

2. **Fortify lunch.** Lunch was usually a whole-grain sandwich, carrot sticks (or other veggies), a granola bar, and a piece of fruit. Trayvon's favorite sandwich was vegan deli slices, mustard, pickles, and lettuce. Sometimes he had a peanut butter and jelly sandwich, or a wrap with hummus and veggies. Since his deli-slice sandwiches are great protein sources, Alejandro suggested exchanging the granola bar for a healthy, plant-based protein bar. This boosted his protein by 10 grams.

3. **Think protein for dinner.** Amy tries to make dinners that appeal to the whole family, and the meals don't always have an obvious protein source. For example, one family favorite is pasta with marinara sauce. Alejandro suggested that Amy use legume-based pasta instead of grain-based pasta and add veggie balls to the meal. He talked about new ways of using tofu, such as the Tasty Tofu Fingers (pages 132–133). By adding at least one concentrated protein source at dinner (such as legumes, legume pasta, tofu, or veggie meats), Amy could add 10–20 grams of protein for each family member.

4. **Incorporate protein into snacks.** Trayvon often stopped at the corner store after school for chips or other salty snacks. Before bed, he had a bowl of cereal with almond milk or a fruit smoothie. Swapping the chips for peanuts or trail mix bumps up protein by 7–10 grams. Using soy instead of almond milk on his cereal and in his smoothie adds 6–7 grams of protein per cup. Adding 3 tablespoons (45 ml) of hemp seeds to his smoothie or cereal provides another 10 grams.

Aisha: Fitting In with Friends

Aisha was born a social butterfly. Fitting in with friends was the most important thing in the world to her. Aisha's resistance to plant-based eating was really resistance to being different from her best friends. Aisha wanted to eat pizza at pizza parties and bring lunches to school that looked like everyone else's. When the family made the shift to plant-based eating, Aisha continued to eat whatever her friends were eating. However, as her perspectives shifted, she was torn. She didn't want to hurt animals, but she didn't want to feel excluded by her circle of friends. She was concerned that if she was too pushy about her dietary choices, her friends might feel uncomfortable or judged. Aisha talked to her parents about her concerns, and they discussed strategies she might use to diffuse challenging social situations. These are Aisha's five favorite strategies:

1. **Get familiar with the menu before going out to eat.** When Aisha's friends planned to eat out, she checked the menu ahead of time. This way, she didn't have to ask if there was anything vegan on the menu. She knew exactly what to order.

2. **Ask and you shall receive.** Aisha found pizza parties really challenging because her friends loved pepperoni or Hawaiian pizza with ham and pineapple. They assumed she would pick the meat off. For a while she did, but it got gross,

especially after her trip to the farm sanctuary. She decided to ask her friends if they would mind if she ordered a small veggie lover's pizza for herself. Her friends were not only supportive, they ordered a large veggie pizza with vegan pepperoni and cheese pizza for everyone to try.

3. **Share delicious food with friends.** Aisha was a budding chef. Her favorite things to make were brownies, cookies, and cakes, but she also experimented with tacos, burgers, pasta, and salads. Aisha loved surprising her friends with treats, and the tasty items always disappeared quickly. She was often asked for recipes and was happy to oblige.

4. **Bring your own food.** When Aisha was going to a sleepover or birthday party, she worried about what she would eat. Aisha asked her friends about the food before the party. She offered to bring whatever might make it easier for the host. If they were making burgers, she would bring a veggie patty. If they were having tacos, she would bring enough veggie meat or black bean filling to share. Aisha found that helping the host was a great way to relieve stress for everyone.

5. **Make your food look yummy.** When Aisha brought leftover beans and rice for lunch one day, some of her friends thought it looked gross. Aisha wanted to do what she could to avoid harsh judgments. Sometimes she brought lunches that looked like everyone else's. But other times she would mix things up with a big colorful salad and crackers with vegan cheese, or hot soup and crusty bread. If she brought beans and rice, she would assemble her dish at school and bring toppings like diced peppers, guacamole, and salsa. She discovered that if she made her food look beautiful, people were more likely to admire her than to tease her.

Lucas: No Beans, Please

Lucas remembered his first bean dish—kidney beans on rice. The beans did not taste like the chicken they usually had on rice. Lucas decided that day that he was not a fan of beans. Whenever Amy served a bean dish, he picked at his food, carefully avoiding the beans. Amy and D'Andre wished that Lucas had not given up on beans so quickly. To make sure he got enough protein, they ended up serving tofu and veggie meats more often. Amy and D'Andre wanted their kids to love eating beans, which are the protein and fiber-rich superstars of the plant kingdom. They were determined to find a way to get Lucas to give beans a chance. They began by teaching him about the long history of legumes all over the world. They showed Lucas pictures of bean dishes—black beans in burritos from Mexico, ful medames with fava beans from Egypt, lentil curry from India, red bean soup from Asia, and hummus from the Middle East. They pointed out a dozen different types of dried beans and five varieties of lentils while shopping. Lucas was happy to help prepare some ethnic recipes. He discovered that fajitas were pretty good, especially with guacamole and vegan cheese. He could not believe how delicious falafels were, and he thought eating edamame right out of the shell was fun. Amy decided to experiment with legume-based burgers and soups, and she scored on all of those fronts. It took a few months of effort, but Lucas became a lover of legumes (and of travel).

Olivia: Cutting Out Cashews

Little Olivia had an allergy to cashews that might have seemed challenging to plant-based parents. Cashews serve as the base for many dairy replacements, such as cheeses, sauces, creams, dessert toppings, ice creams, yogurts, and milks. Some family favorites were cashew based, so it was quite a blow when they discovered Olivia's allergy. Amy found that sunflower seeds made a good replacement in sauces, cheeses, and creams. For some recipes, skinned almonds also did the trick.

Allergies to nuts, seeds, soy, and other legumes can be challenging for anyone. Fortunately, there are many ways to put together a healthy diet.

You can rest assured that plant protein is perfect for your children and teens. Get creative with your protein, and be sure to include your children in the selection and preparation of meals and snacks. For tips on boosting protein intake, see pages 105–107. For suggested menus, see pages 108–109.

References for this chapter are online at https://plant-poweredprotein.com/references.

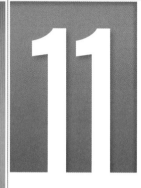

Protein for Plant-Based Athletes

Plant-based athletes are rising to the top of their games. Many of these athletes find improvements in both performance and recovery when they swap animal-based protein for plant-based protein. Among the most inspiring is ultra-endurance mountain biker Sonya Looney. Here is her story:

I always thought that getting diseases like cancer, heart disease, and high blood pressure was something that happened to everyone as they got older. As a professional athlete, I was focused on reducing processed foods and eating as many whole foods as possible. When I watched the *Forks Over Knives* documentary in 2013 and learned that animal products are linked to many lifestyle diseases, I decided to switch to a whole-food, plant-based diet. I was nervous about how this would impact my performance. By 2013, I was competing at the top level of the ultra-endurance racing circuit (consisting of single-day, 100-mile mountain bike races, seven-day mountain bike stage races, and 24-hour racing). I was worried I wouldn't get the nutrients and protein I needed if I completely cut out meat, dairy, and eggs. I didn't know many people who were plant based and competing at the top level in endurance sports. I gradually shifted my eating habits over the course of a few months to make sure I could still train hard, recover, and race well. *Becoming Vegan: Comprehensive Edition* by Brenda Davis and Vesanto Melina was the book I used as my guide.

Something unexpected happened after I changed my diet. I got faster and stronger. I was worried about getting weaker and slower and the opposite happened! I noticed that I could recover faster from my workouts, and I suffered from way less overuse injuries caused by inflammation. My body composition also changed to being leaner while maintaining muscle mass and power. Over the next year, my race results also improved! I went from trying to fight for the last spot on the podium to competing for the win (and often winning races!). In 2015, I was crowned World Champion in 24-Hour Racing, and I continue to win and set course records at some of the most prestigious races in the world! I've raced in more than 25 countries to date.

Occasionally, I would do a three-day check and keep a log of what I was eating and make sure I was getting enough protein. I noticed that I did not have any trouble meeting my protein targets because I included legumes (including tofu and tempeh), whole grains, nuts/seeds, and veggies with each meal. I was never a fan of protein powders, even before I changed my diet. It's still not something that I feel is necessary. During longer races or particularly grueling training blocks, I do include a branched-chain amino acid supplement. I've also used beta-alanine and leucine, but they are not regular supplements. The sports drink I use during competition and training includes branched-chain amino acids to slow muscle breakdown, and I've found that to be helpful. I love having the confidence that the food I'm eating not only supports my health and performance potential, but it leaves a much smaller carbon footprint and reduces harm to others. I've done multiple blood panels over the years and my numbers are consistently in the healthy range.

Protein is the macronutrient that reigns supreme in the minds of most athletes. When athletes shift to plant-based diets, their coaches, trainers, and teammates worry about how protein needs will be met. In this chapter, we examine these concerns and provide practical guidelines for meeting protein needs with plants.

WHY PROTEIN IS IMPORTANT FOR ATHLETES

Protein is required for building, repairing, and preserving muscle mass. It also plays a critical role in the integrity and function of non-muscle tissue, such as bones and tendons. A single session of resistance or aerobic training leads to an increase in muscle protein synthesis for at least 24 hours. This muscle gain is supported by dietary protein intake over this time. Protein-deficient diets can compromise structure and function in athletes, resulting in reduced performance.

How Much Protein Athletes Need

The adult recommended dietary allowance for protein is 0.8 grams per kilogram of body weight (see chapter 2). The recommended dietary allowance is considered sufficient for people who are sedentary, lightly active, or moderately active. Four groups have established protein recommendations for athletes in official position statements: the Academy of Nutrition and Dietetics, Dietitians of Canada, and the American College of Sports Medicine in their 2016 position on nutrition and athletic performance; and the International Society of Sports Nutrition in its 2017 position on protein and exercise.

Table 11.1 (page 88) summarizes protein recommendations for athletes and the general population. Protein needs are provided in grams per kilogram of body weight per day. For athletes who are plant based, adding 10 percent to these recommendations compensates for the reduced digestibility of protein from whole plant foods. This addition is not required for plant-based athletes who regularly consume animal products, such as milk, eggs, or fish. It also isn't

TABLE 11.1. Recommended protein intakes for active adults and for athletes

RECOMMENDATIONS	ADULTS INCLUDING ACTIVE PEOPLE (RDA[1])	ATHLETES (AND[2], DC[3], ACSM[4])	PLANT-BASED ATHLETES (AND[2], DC[3], ACSM[4]) +10%	ATHLETES (ISSN[5])	PLANT-BASED ATHLETES (ISSN[5]) +10%
Total protein (grams per kilogram of weight per day)	0.8	1.2–2.0	1.3–2.2	1.4–2.0	1.5–2.2
Total essential amino acids	214 mg/kg/day	10 grams 0–2 hours after exercise	11 grams 0–2 hours after exercise	10–12 grams every 3–4 hours	11–13 grams every 3–4 hours
Branched-chain amino acids (grams)	5–8*			10–14*	11–15*
Leucine	42 mg/kg/day			700–3,000 mg every 3–4 hours	770–3,300 mg every 3–4 hours
Timing of total protein intake		15–25 grams or 0.3 g/kg 0–2 hours after exercise and every 3–5 hours	17–28 grams or 0.33 g/kg 0–2 hours after exercise and every 3–5 hours	20–40 grams or 0.25 g/kg every 3–4 hours	22–44 grams or 0.28 g/kg every 3–4 hours

[1]Recommended dietary allowance
[2]Academy of Nutrition and Dietetics
[3]Dietitians of Canada
[4]American College of Sports Medicine
[5]International Society of Sports Nutrition

*Recommended dietary allowance for branched-chain amino acids is 86 mg/kg/day for adults. For adults weighing 132–198 pounds (60–90 kg), the range would be 5–8 grams.

necessary for people who regularly consume very low-fiber, plant-protein foods, such as tofu, soy milk, veggie meat, or protein powders.

As you can see in table 11.1, above, athletes need more protein than the general population. The International Society of Sports Nutrition suggests intakes of 2.3–3.1 grams per kilogram of body weight per day to maximize muscle retention in resistance-trained athletes during periods of low-calorie intakes. An example of this would be a bodybuilder who is cutting calories to get as lean as possible for competition. Meeting these targets is not as difficult as you might expect, as most athletes eat a lot of food, and a lot of protein.

Can Athletes Get Enough Leucine and Other Branched-Chain Amino Acids from Plants?

The answer is yes, providing that protein from a variety of sources is consumed and the recommended protein intakes for athletes are met. The reason for the concern is that branched-chain amino acids are needed for building and maintaining muscle and are most concentrated in animal products. The three branched-chain amino acids—leucine, isoleucine, and valine—stimulate protein synthesis in skeletal muscle and other tissues. They inhibit muscle loss and improve recovery. Of the three, leucine plays the most important role in stimulating protein synthesis. However, all three help to promote muscle gains and minimize muscle breakdown. Plant-based athletes can get enough leucine and other branched-chain amino acids from legumes, soy foods, wheat gluten (seitan), seeds, nuts, and grains. See table 11.1 (page 88) for recommended intakes of leucine and branched-chain amino acids. Precise needs vary with age, body size, metabolism, state of health, and type and intensity of training. See table 3.1 (pages 24–25) for the leucine content of common foods, and see chapter 3, pages 22–23, for further information on branched-chain amino acids.

Is the Timing of Protein Intake Important for Maximizing Beneficial Effects for Athletes?

Yes, the timing of protein intake is important. Muscle protein synthesis occurs only with sufficient food. In a fasting state, protein balance is negative and muscle gains cannot be achieved.

To maximize muscle protein synthesis, the International Society of Sports Nutrition recommends eating every 3–4 hours throughout the day. The Academy of Nutrition and Dietetics, Dietitians of Canada, and the American College of Sports Medicine recommend eating every 3–5 hours throughout the day. The International Society of Sports Nutrition suggests that the best time to consume protein relative to workouts is based on individual tolerance. It adds that the timing of ingestion is less of a priority than total daily intake. The Academy of Nutrition and Dietetics, Dietitians of Canada, and the American College of Sports Medicine suggest that increases in strength and muscle mass appear greatest when protein is consumed 0–2 hours after exercise. Eating a protein-rich snack before bed has demonstrated benefits for resistance training. It can help to meet daily protein targets and provides a stimulus for muscle growth. For recommended amounts of protein to include with meals and snacks, see table 11.1 (page 88).

Is Plant Protein Sufficient for Building Muscle Mass and Increasing Strength?

Yes, studies have shown that plant protein is just as effective as animal protein for muscle protein synthesis. A 2018 meta-analysis reported that soy protein produced about the same muscle and strength gains as whey protein. A 2017 study of almost 3,000 adults with different dietary patterns found that muscle mass and quadriceps strength increased with total protein intake. People in the lowest quartile (one-quarter of the group) of protein intake had the lowest strength. Protein from plants and animals was equally effective in promoting muscle mass and strength.

Are There Advantages to Eating Plant Protein over Animal Protein?

Yes, plant proteins offer a number of advantages for athletes. Choosing plant-based over animal-based protein-rich foods reduces the risk of chronic disease and obesity. What many athletes fail to realize is that the benefits of plant protein extend to performance as well. These are some of the key advantages:

- **Plant-protein foods improve circulation.** Protein-rich plant foods can reduce plaque buildup in the arteries. They lower blood viscosity and increase arterial elasticity. This improves blood flow. Better blood flow means more oxygen and nutrients to the muscles and better elimination of metabolic waste products.

- **Plant-protein foods reduce inflammation.** Whole plant foods are rich in anti-inflammatory compounds. These foods are our primary sources of protective phytochemicals, antioxidants, vitamin E, and healthful fats. Animal products tend to have pro-inflammatory effects. Chronic inflammation can cause tissue damage, pain, and fatigue. This can compromise oxygen delivery and hinder athletic performance.

- **Plant-protein foods reduce oxidative stress.** Physical training increases the production of free radicals, which can damage body tissues. When the body manufactures more free radicals than it can neutralize with antioxidants, oxidative stress occurs. Exercise-induced oxidative stress can damage body tissues, resulting in reduced performance and recovery. Athletes need a steady supply of antioxidants from foods. The most potent antioxidants are concentrated in plant foods. These include vitamin E, vitamin C, provitamin A carotenoids, selenium, and many phytochemicals.

- **Plant-protein foods support a healthy gut microbiome.** A healthy, diverse microbiome is sustained by fiber, which provides food for the gut bacteria. High-protein plant foods, such as legumes (beans, peas, and lentils), are loaded with fiber, while animal products have none. A healthy gut microbiome has a fundamental role in metabolism, endocrine function, and immune response. It helps with the delivery of water, nutrients, and hormones during exercise.

- **Plant-protein foods promote lean bodies.** Plant foods deliver fewer calories for any given volume of food, which may help to explain why plant-based eaters are typically leaner. Lower levels of body fat are associated with improved aerobic capacity and better endurance.

- **Most plant-protein foods help build glycogen stores.** Endurance performance depends on stores of glycogen, which is the body's backup source of fuel derived from carbohydrates. Carbohydrates are also the preferred fuel for our brains. Plant foods, such as legumes, provide high-quality carbohydrates, while meat is devoid of carbohydrates.

Ensuring Ample Protein from Plants

Plant-based athletes who fall short on protein are those who restrict their energy intake or who eat few legumes and meat alternatives. Insufficient protein can compromise the maintenance, repair, and synthesis of skeletal muscle. While it is not necessary to eat specific combinations of plant proteins at each meal, it is important to consume protein-rich foods. At some meals or snacks, it may help to have a smoothie with added branched-chain amino acids or vegan protein powder. Table 11.2, below, provides examples of how you might boost protein throughout the day. See pages 105–107 for our top 10 tips for boosting daily protein intake. Table 4.1 (pages 32–39) provides the protein content of common foods.

TABLE 11.2. Examples of simple protein boosts

INSTEAD OF:	CHOOSE:	PROTEIN GAINED* (GRAMS)
BREAKFAST		
1½ cups (375 ml) cornflakes 1 cup (250 m) almond milk 1 banana	1 cup (250 ml) Gorilla Granola (page 127–128) 1 cup (250 ml) soy milk 1 banana	24
LUNCH		
4 cups (1 L) green salad 2 tablespoons (30 ml) Italian dressing 1 whole-grain bagel 2 tablespoons (30 ml) plant-based cream cheese	4 cups (1 L) green salad ¼ cup (60 ml) Lemon-Tahini Protein-Plus Dressing (page 148) 4 ounces (120 g) Tasty Tofu Fingers (page 132–133) or 1¼ cups (310 ml) beans 3 tablespoons (45 ml) pumpkin seeds 1 whole-grain bagel 2 tablespoons (30 ml) plant-based cream cheese	34
DINNER		
2 cups (500 ml) wheat pasta 1 cup (250 ml) marinara sauce 2 cups (500 ml) steamed broccoli	2 cups (500 ml) black bean pasta 1 cup (250 ml) marinara sauce 2 cups (500 ml) steamed broccoli	26
SNACKS		
3 cups (750 ml) green smoothie with banana, blueberries, kale, and water	3 cups (750 ml) Green Power Smoothie (page 124) with optional soft tofu	26
2 ounces (60 g) pretzels	2 ounces (60 g) peanuts	8
1 granola bar	1 vegan power bar	12
4 oatmeal cookies (packaged)	4 Double-Chocolate Surprise Cookies (page 135)	9

*Protein gains will vary slightly with brands selected. Source: US Department of Agriculture, Agricultural Research Service. FoodData Central, 2019. fdc.nal.usda.gov.

Do Plant-Based Athletes Benefit by
Taking Protein and Amino Acid Supplements?

When it comes to athletic performance, ensuring a high-quality diet is a top priority. Our food guide and menus on pages 105–109 will assist you in this task. Plant-based athletes may wonder if they would gain a competitive edge by adding protein or amino acid supplements to their daily regime, but that may not always be necessary. While supplements may augment performance for some athletes, dietary adjustments are often sufficient. However, let's review the protein and amino acid supplements that are of greatest interest to plant-based athletes. Check with your health-care provider before adding supplements.

Beta-alanine. Beta-alanine is a nonessential, nonprotein amino acid, which is an amino acid that is not used to make protein. It is one of two amino acids (the other being histidine) needed for the formation of carnosine. Carnosine helps to increase performance by reducing lactic acid buildup in muscles. Carnosine is present only in animal products, with meat and poultry being the main sources. Beta-alanine supplements increase muscle carnosine concentrations. Studies suggest beta-alanine can increase athletic performance in high-intensity training. Muscle levels of carnosine are lower in plant-based eaters. Beta-alanine supplements may be more effective for plant-based athletes than for meat-eating athletes, although research is lacking. Vegan beta-alanine is available. Minimal safety concerns have been reported for doses of up to 6.4 grams per day for up to 24 weeks. Beta-alanine supplementation may cause a prickling or burning sensation in the face, neck, back of the hands, and upper trunk.

Creatine. Creatine is among the most popular supplements for athletes, particularly strength athletes. It is one of the few performance supplements with demonstrated effects in clinical trials. Creatine supplementation reduces fatigue during short bursts of high-intensity activities. It has also been shown to improve strength and muscle mass. Creatine is of special interest to plant-based athletes because it is found only in meat—including our own flesh. The human body manufactures about 1 gram of creatine per day from precursor amino acids. Creatine synthesis is increased when plant-based diets are consumed. While internal production compensates to some extent for differences in dietary intakes, blood and tissue creatine concentrations are lower among plant-based eaters than omnivores. Plant-based athletes may enjoy greater benefits from taking creatine than omnivores. Synthetically produced, plant-based creatine is available. According to the National Institutes of Health, doses of 20 grams per day (divided into four portions of 5 grams each) for up to 7 days, followed by 3–5 grams a day for up to 12 weeks, are safe for adults. The most common adverse effects are fluid retention, cramps, nausea, and diarrhea. Creatine is best avoided by people with kidney disease. The effects of long-term creatine supplementation are not known.

Branched-chain amino acids and leucine. For endurance athletes, studies have not shown enhanced performance with branched-chain amino acid supplements. However, they may delay feelings of fatigue and help with mental focus. For strength athletes, short-term studies found gains in muscle mass and strength with 10–14 grams of supplemental branched-chain amino acids per day. Branched-chain amino acid supplements may reduce muscle damage and promote muscle-protein synthesis, decreasing muscle soreness. Sufficient branched-chain amino acids, including leucine, can be obtained from plant-based diets. However, for people whose diets fall short of protein, a protein powder or a dedicated branched-chain amino acid supplement may be of value. If a branched-chain amino acid supplement is used, opt for one with a ratio of 2:1:1 leucine, isoleucine, and valine (twice as much leucine as isoleucine or valine). An intake of at least 200 milligrams per kilogram of body weight per day for 10 days, starting at least 7 days prior to intense exercise, may help limit muscle damage from intense activity. Branched-chain amino acid supplements of up to 20 grams a day in divided doses appear safe. For leucine, an upper limit of 500 milligrams per kilogram per day or 35 grams per day has been suggested for healthy adult men. Similar recommendations have not been made for women.

Protein supplements. Protein supplements, such as powders and bars, are the most popular supplements used by fitness enthusiasts. For people who meet recommended protein intakes, these supplements do little to boost performance or muscle gains. However, for athletes who have difficulty meeting protein needs from food, these supplements can be of value. This is especially true for people doing short bursts of intense training or who are trying to lose body fat for competition.

What Are the Best Choices in Protein Powders for Vegans?

Plant-based athletes have protein powder options based on soy, pea, corn, potato, hemp, and rice proteins. When selecting a supplement, look for one that contains a mix of plant proteins. This helps boost protein quality, including the branched-chain amino acid content. Surprisingly, corn protein tops the list of plant-based proteins for leucine, with potato protein coming a close second. Although potatoes are low in protein, extracted potato protein has an impressive amino acid profile. Next, look at the ingredient list. Be wary of protein powders that contain fillers, additives, preservatives, sugars, thickeners, and artificial colors. Some products contain environmental contaminants, such as lead, arsenic, cadmium, mercury, BPA, and pesticides. Look for a third-party certification stamp on the label to ensure the product has been screened for safety. The United States Anti-Doping Agency recognizes NSF's Certified for Sport as the best label to ensure the lowest risk from contaminants in supplements.

Can Athletes Get Too Much Protein?

Yes, it is possible to get too much protein, but you don't have to worry about getting too much protein if you obtain it from whole plant foods. However, if you include large amounts of extracted proteins, such as protein powders, in your daily diet, it is possible to overdo it. It is easier to consume too much protein on an omnivorous diet because meat, poultry, and fish are free of carbohydrates. Instead, all their calories come from protein and fat. Plant foods contain a balance of all three macronutrients. High animal-protein intakes are associated with an increased risk of chronic diseases, including kidney stones, gout, some cancers, liver disorders, and coronary artery disease. The critical question is, How much protein is too much? For most individuals, an intake of 2 grams of protein per kilogram of body weight is considered a safe upper limit. Some elite athletes and bodybuilders may need slightly more during periods of intense training.

References for this chapter are online at https://plant-poweredprotein.com/references.

Energetic Elders

We are heading into the "Silver Tsunami." In 1950, 8 percent of the North American population was aged 65 and over. It is now more than double that and will almost triple to 22 percent by 2050. The number of centenarians will have increased more than 100-fold in less than a century. Some of us are moving forward with our walking sticks and wheelchairs—and many are striding forth with vigor and vitality.

Much more than years of ill health, retirement can bring decades of vibrant well-being. Chapters 6 and 7 showed that by choosing a plant-based diet, we can significantly reduce our risk of chronic disease.

Harvard-based research followed more than 100,000 Americans for over two decades. It found that by making four or five lifestyle choices from the age of 50, we can expect to live well into our 80s (or longer) instead of just into our 70s. Furthermore, these added years will be less burdened by chronic diseases, such as diabetes, cardiovascular disease, and cancer. The following lifestyle choices increase longevity:

- Maintaining an optimal weight (BMI or waist-to-hip ratio).
- Getting at least one-half hour of moderate or vigorous exercise a day.
- Not smoking.
- Minimizing alcohol.
- Getting seven or more hours of sleep.
- Having a supportive network of family or friends.
- Looking for other health-oriented adults your age who live nearby, by searching online for vegetarian, vegan, or plant-based groups, activities, or restaurants.
- Using online dating to look for someone whose interests are complementary, and then sharing cooking skills and enthusiasm.
- Basing your diet on unprocessed and lightly processed whole plant foods such as fruits, vegetables, legumes, whole grains, nuts, and seeds and minimizing

intake of highly processed foods with added fat, sugar, and salt, red and processed meat, and alcohol.

For many adults, getting enough protein is not an issue. But for seniors, whether plant based or nonvegan, it can become a challenge. You may have heard that limiting food intake may help you to live longer. It is true that as we age, our caloric requirements decrease, and it is good to maintain a healthy body weight. Yet protein needs increase, rather than decrease, as we age. So we need more bang (protein) for our buck (calories). Proteins play a vital role in the structure, function, and regulation of our tissues and organs (see pages 7–8). In this chapter we will focus on protein's role in maintaining bone health and muscle mass.

KEEPING BONES STRONG: CALCIUM, VITAMIN D, PROTEIN, AND EXERCISE

When we think of bone structure, our thoughts often turn to calcium. However, four pillars support our bone health:

1. A key to strong bones, protein provides the matrix in which calcium and other minerals are embedded.

2. Calcium provides structure and hardness. The recommended dietary allowance is 1,200 milligrams of calcium per day for women 50-plus years old and men 70-plus, and 1,000 milligrams for men 51–70.

3. Vitamin D improves absorption and retention of calcium. Our intake should maintain serum 25-hydroxyvitamin D levels of at least 20 nanograms per milliliter (50 nanomoles per liter).

4. Weight-bearing exercise stimulates bones to hold on to their minerals. Muscle strength also protects us against falling and breaking bones.

A past theory proposed that high protein intakes could lead to calcium losses through the kidneys and thereby weaken bones. This can be true with high intakes of meat or of protein powders, especially when calcium intakes are low. However, we have no evidence of such calcium losses happening with plant foods. Instead, we find that eating protein-rich plant foods can increase our intestinal absorption of calcium and stimulate the hormone IGF-1, which manages the effects of growth hormone in our bodies. IGF-1 is a protein builder and supports bone health. One of the benefits of getting sufficient protein from plants is that it boosts IGF-1 production, without being excessive. With high-protein, animal-based diets, IGF-1 levels can rise enough to increase the risk of some cancers.

MUSCLE MASS AND SARCOPENIA

With age, people typically experience a gradual decline in muscle mass and strength. Every decade after the age of 30, adults may lose up to 1–5 percent of their muscle mass and greater losses of strength. This rate of loss doubles after age 70. Some people lose muscle mass and strength more quickly and develop a condition called sarcopenia. Normally muscle cells have continual turnover. With age, there can be more muscle cell breakdown than building. Sarcopenia's causes include lower intakes of protein (along with other nutrients), physical inactivity, inflammation, and changes with hormones. The prevalence of sarcopenia is 5–13 percent for those in their 60s and higher in nursing homes and with increased age.

Yet our muscle strength and mass are keys to staying active and independent. Sarcopenia can result in poor quality of life, disability, and chronic disease. The strength of our grip or leg muscles, our walking speed, and other measures of physical function are used as indicators of sarcopenia.

Adequate intakes of protein and of the protein-building amino acid leucine are linked with improved physical performance and protection against muscle wasting. For more on leucine-rich foods, see chapter 3, pages 24–25. It is important to have your overall diet support the renewal of muscle cells, based on the food guide on pages 102–104. This includes fruits and vegetables for protective antioxidants and vitamins D and B_{12}. Keep your lab values of vitamin D in the recommended range—a minimum of 20 nanograms per milliliter (50 nanomoles per liter). Although exposure of skin to sunlight can result in vitamin D production by the body, in most geographic regions this requires some vitamin D supplementation, with necessary amounts varying from one individual to another. Also, serum vitamin B_{12} levels of 300 picomoles per liter (400 picograms/ml) or more can help protect muscle mass and strength in older people.

HIGHER RECOMMENDED INTAKES OF PROTEIN FOR SENIORS

To maintain or to regain lean body mass (muscle), 1–1.2 grams of protein per kilogram of healthy body weight is considered to be optimal for people aged 65 years and older. For people on plant-based diets, we recommend 1.1–1.3 grams of protein per kilogram of healthy body weight per day. Each meal should include at least 700 milligrams of leucine for protein synthesis.

BUILDING PROTEIN-RICH MEALS AND SNACKS

Since muscle synthesis is improved for a few hours after consuming protein, it is wise to have protein-rich foods at each meal and for snacks. For example, choose from those listed below. A meal or snack providing at least 20 grams of protein is recommended right after exercise, and it should deliver at least 700 milligrams of leucine. For more on exercise, see pages 99–100.

Breakfast:

- Sip a Green Power Smoothie (page 124); sometimes try the Protein Boosters listed.
- Enjoy Gorilla Granola (pages 127–128) or Powered-Up Overnight Oats (page 125) with soy milk.
- Feast on Golden Scrambled Tofu (page 129).
- Eat two or three slices of toast, each with 1 tablespoon (15 ml) of peanut butter; 3 tablespoons of peanut butter will deliver 20 grams of protein plus 1,000 milligrams of leucine.
- Use soy milk in your coffee or tea; 1 cup (250 ml) delivers 6–8 grams of protein and 622 milligrams of leucine. If you look at the labels on other nondairy milks, you will find most to be much lower in protein. Fortified or enriched soy milk provides calcium and vitamin D as well.

Snacks:

- Keep Tasty Tofu Fingers (pages 132–133) handy in the fridge for instant munching, hot or cold.
- Chia Pudding (page 134) and cookies (pages 135–137) are helpful and tasty sweet treats.

Lunch or Dinner:

- Browse the recipes in chapter 15 for some delicious choices. See the nutritional analysis with each recipe.
- Also see the tips in chapter 13 and table 13.1 (page 103).
- For quick protein solutions, explore the veggie meats section of your local supermarket. That area may have expanded greatly since you last looked. You will find a wide range of plant-based sausages, deli slices, burgers, ground round, and more that taste like the less health-supportive animal products they replace. Labels show the wealth of protein that these easy-to-use products deliver.

Recommended Protein and Leucine Intakes for Special Health Conditions

People with acute or chronic diseases may need 1.2–1.5 grams of protein per kilogram of healthy body weight and even more in some cases. For people with sarcopenia, each meal should provide 25–30 grams of protein and include 2.5–2.8 grams of leucine. Meeting these goals while rebuilding muscle mass is easier with small amounts of supplemental leucine or branched-chain amino acids.

In contrast, people with severe kidney disease need to limit protein, as directed by their health-care provider. For these individuals, switching from animal products to plant-based foods has been shown to delay the progression of the disease and reduce mortality.

ANIMAL PROTEIN OR PLANT PROTEIN?

People think of meat and cheese as protein foods, but in truth they could be viewed as fat foods, as most of their calories are from the fat category. When these products are featured prominently in the diet, they can contribute to the accumulation of visceral fat in and around our vital organs. This fat emits molecules that promote inflammation. Avoiding excess fat, excess calories, and animal products will increase longevity. A Harvard study found that replacing 3 percent of our calories from animal protein with plant protein can help us live longer. For example, we can reduce our risk of dying by 20 percent by replacing each egg or two slices of bacon eaten daily with one of these: a falafel patty, ¼ cup (60 ml) of black beans, 2 teaspoons (10 ml) of peanut butter, or 3 tablespoons (45 ml) of tofu. In addition, replacing animal protein with plant protein reduces the risk of heart disease, type 2 diabetes, and some cancers. One study also found those eating vegetarian (near vegan) diets had a 38 percent lower risk of dementia. An Adventist Health Study among 51,082 participants found a marked tendency to consume less meat, poultry, and fish as people age.

EXERCISE: A KEY TO MUSCLE BUILDING

Muscle building does not occur with good nutrition alone. At least 30–60 minutes a day of exercise can help fend off and even reverse the decline in muscle size and strength. It's good to do a mix of activities, including resistance or weight training, aerobic exercise, endurance, interval training, activities for balance, and stretching. For people in their 90s, a study showed that a two-month program of resistance training nearly doubled the muscle strength of participants and increased their walking speed by 50 percent. It's never too late to start.

Physical activity leads to dozens of positive changes in metabolism, circulation, muscles, bones, and the nerves that connect the brain with muscles. Exercise increases the length of telomeres—the protective caps on DNA strands that are linked with longevity. It reduces the number of muscle cells that have stopped dividing and increases the number of stem cells that renew muscle. Exercised muscle contains more and better mitochondria than sedentary muscle. Being active may result in the destruction and rebuilding of aging collagen, meaning that stiff fibers are replaced with fresh new ones. Considered as a whole, our muscles are the biggest organ in the body. This is significant because static (unmoving) muscle tends to promote inflammation, whereas active muscle reduces inflammation. Exercise can burn the fat that produces inflammatory molecules, thereby reducing inflammation. In these ways, exercise slows the aging process and even decreases our risk of cognitive decline or dementia.

PRACTICAL TIPS AND RESOURCES FOR INCREASING PROTEIN INTAKE

Nutrition for Care Facilities and Home Support

The Vegetarian Resource Group (vrg.org/seniors) provides resources for nursing homes and assisted living facilities. It lists a four-week menu cycle for Meals on Wheels America. Having the overworked chef in a small facility provide simple, plant-protein entrées for a resident may take some communication and help. Yet we have seen it work.

Affordable Protein and a Better World

Beans (there are more than 20 types), peas, and lentils are very affordable ways to get protein. They should be cooked well (see pages 119–120). To help the intestines adjust, start with small portions. Cook a big batch of dried legumes and freeze them in meal-size portions. The protein and minerals in beans, peas, and lentils survive cooking and canning very well. Tofu is a great protein option that is soft and easy to chew and can be seasoned in a wide variety of ways.

Overall, research shows that diets higher in legumes, nuts, seeds, whole grains, vegetables, and fruits and lower in animal products support human health and environmental sustainability. So, in creating your plant protein-rich diet, you are not only treating yourself to better health, but you also are treating your children, grandchildren, and future generations to a better world.

References for this chapter are online at https://plant-poweredprotein.com/references.

The Plant-Based Plate, Tips, and Menus

13

The Plant-Based Plate can help you create an eating plan that works for you and every family member (from age one and beyond). This guide features five food groups: vegetables, fruits, grains, legumes, and nuts and seeds. When planning meals, try to include something from all or most food groups. Of course, specific choices will vary from day to day. Table 13.1 on page 103 shows a suggested minimum number of servings to be consumed during the day, based on the nutrient contribution from each food group. These serving sizes are suitable for everyone nine years of age or older. For toddlers aged one to three, serving sizes are halved, and for young children four to eight, serving sizes are about three-quarters those of older children and adults. It's not difficult to achieve the recommended servings, as the serving sizes are small. Don't worry if you're not meeting all the targets every day. Instead, focus on eating a variety of these nutrient-dense foods. In the Plant-Based Plate illustration (page 102), the items in the small plate labeled Other Essentials are explained below. For more details about choices rich in calcium and protein, see page 103.

OTHER ESSENTIALS

Even if you consume the suggested servings from each food group, some important nutrients can fall short. These are "other essentials."

For omega-3 fatty acids, include at least one of the following daily:

- 2 tablespoons (30 ml) ground flaxseeds or chia seeds
- ¼ cup (60 ml) hemp seeds
- ⅓ cup (85 ml) walnuts
- 1½ teaspoons (7 ml) flaxseed oil

Each of these examples provides about 3.2 grams of ALA (alpha-linolenic acid), which is enough for the average man and more than enough for the average woman, who needs only 2.2 grams. An additional supplement of 200–300 milligrams of vegan DHA (docosahexaenoic acid) two to three times a week is optional.

FIGURE 13.1. The plant-based plate.

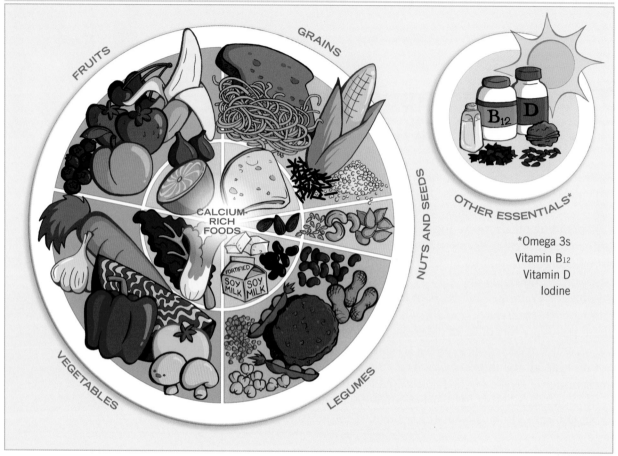

For vitamin B$_{12}$, include at least one of the following:

- A daily supplement that provides at least 50 micrograms of vitamin B$_{12}$.
- Twice a week, a supplement that provides at least 1,000 micrograms of vitamin B$_{12}$.
- Three servings over the course of a day of vitamin B$_{12}$-fortified foods, such as nondairy milks, vegan meat alternatives, or breakfast cereals, each fortified with a total of 2.4 micrograms of vitamin B$_{12}$ per serving or 100 percent of the Daily Value (check the label). Two teaspoons (10 ml or 5 g) of Red Star Nutritional Yeast Vegetarian Support Formula can qualify as one of these servings.

For vitamin D, take a supplement, eat fortified foods, get daily exposure to sunlight, or use a combination of these (page 104):

TABLE 13.1. The plant-based plate: Daily guide for healthful eating

FOOD GROUP (NUMBER OF SERVINGS SUGGESTED*)	FOODS INCLUDED (SERVING SIZES*)	CALCIUM-RICH CHOICES	PROTEIN-RICH CHOICES (GRAMS OF PROTEIN PER SERVING***)
Vegetables (5 or more servings) Choose a rainbow of colors.	½ cup (125 ml) raw or cooked vegetables 1 cup (250 ml) raw leafy vegetables ½ cup (125 ml) vegetable juice	Bok choy, broccoli, collard greens, kale, mustard greens, napa cabbage, or okra** Calcium-fortified tomato or vegetable juice	Fresh peas (4) Hubbard squash (3) Spinach, cooked (2.7) Corn (2.4)
Fruits (4 or more servings) Go for variety!	1 medium fruit ½ cup (125 ml) fruit or fruit juice ¼ cup (60 ml) dried fruit	Calcium-fortified fruit juice Dried figs Oranges	Guava, durian, mango (2) Avocado (1.5)
Legumes (3 or more servings) Include with meals and snacks.	½ cup (125 ml) cooked beans, peas, lentils, tofu, or tempeh 1 cup (250 ml) peas or sprouted lentils or peas 1 cup (250 ml) soy or pea milk ¼ cup (60 ml) peanuts 2 tablespoons (30 ml) peanut butter 2 ounces (60 g) vegan meat alternative	Calcium-fortified soy milk, pea milk or soy yogurt Edamame, soybeans, black beans, or white beans Tofu with added calcium	Firm tofu or tempeh (17–20) Soybeans, cooked (17) Veggie meat (15) Edamame (11) Peanuts (10) Adzuki beans, lentils, split peas (9) Other beans (7–8)
Grains (3 or more servings) Choose mostly whole grains.	3 ounces (90 g) seitan ½ cup (125 ml) cooked grain or pasta ½ cup (125 ml) sprouted grains 1 ounce (30 g) ready-to-eat cereal, bread, flatbread, or crackers	Calcium-fortified oat milk Calcium-fortified cereal Calcium-fortified tortilla	Seitan (16) Amaranth, kamut, spelt (5) Quinoa (4) Pasta (4–5) Other grains (2–3)
Nuts and seeds (1 or more servings) Include an omega-3-rich choice.	¼ cup (60 ml) nuts or seeds 2 tablespoons (30 ml) nut or seed butter	Calcium-fortified nut or seed milks Almonds, almond butter Chia seeds Sesame seeds, tahini	Hemp seeds (14) Hemp hearts (13) Pumpkin seeds (10) Almonds (8) Chia and sunflower seeds (7) Nut and seed butters (6–7) Most other nuts and seeds (5–6)

*Serving sizes are for people nine years of age or older. For toddlers one to three years old, servings are half of the size listed; for children four to eight, servings are three-quarters of the size listed.

**Beet greens, spinach, and Swiss chard are high in calcium, but because the calcium is poorly absorbed from these greens (due to high oxalate content), they are not listed.

***Serving sizes are shown in the Foods Included column.

- Supplements or fortified foods. The recommended dietary allowance for vitamin D is 15 micrograms (600 IU) for people up to 70 years old and 20 micrograms (800 IU) for people older than 70. Fortified foods, such as non-dairy milks, can supply part of this. Significantly more, in supplement form, may be needed to reach optimal serum 25-hydroxy vitamin D levels (at least 20 nanograms per milliliter/50 nanomoles per liter and more may be better).
- Exposing the face and forearms to sunlight between 10 a.m. and 3 p.m. for 10–30 minutes at certain latitudes and in warm seasons may stimulate the body to reach optimal vitamin D levels. It is important to avoid excessive exposure to ultraviolet light.

For iodine, take a multivitamin-mineral supplement that contains iodine or consume about ½ teaspoon (2 ml) of iodized salt for the daily recommended intake of 150 micrograms of iodine for adults (slightly lower intakes for children; slightly higher intakes during pregnancy and lactation). Sea vegetables, such as kelp, also contain iodine, though the amount of iodine in these can vary greatly and even reach toxic levels. Read product labels to see whether iodine is listed.

Practical Pointers

To ensure consumption of sufficient nutrients and protective phytochemicals—and to make meals appealing—include a wide variety of plant foods on a daily basis. Plan meals using the Plant-Based Plate (page 102):

- Fill at least half of your plate (or a day's intake) with an assortment of vegetables and fruits.
- Fill at least one-quarter of your plate with legumes or other protein-rich choices.
- Select whole grains (such as barley, quinoa, or spelt berries) or minimally processed options, such as bulgur, steel-cut oats, or rolled oats.
- Limit intakes of added fats, oils, and sugars, if used. Whole foods, such as seeds, nuts, and avocados, should be the primary sources of fat, and fruits the primary sources of sugar.
- Monitor sodium consumption. Use of ready-to-eat processed foods can result in high sodium intakes; check product labels and balance intakes with fresh, unprocessed items.
- Aim for an hour of physical activity each day for energy balance and overall health. Daily exercise helps to maintain muscle strength, bone density, physical balance, and mental well-being.
- Stay hydrated. Make water your beverage of choice. Herbal teas and vegetable juices can add variety. Steer clear of sweetened beverages.

TOP 10 TIPS FOR PILING ON PLANT PROTEIN

T here are many ways to boost protein in your meals and snacks. Here are our top 10 suggestions that are suitable for every stage of life. See pages 97–98 in chapter 12 for additional ideas and page 91 in chapter 11 for practical swaps you can make to boost protein in your meals and snacks.

1. **Use high-protein nondairy milks.** Compare the protein content of your non-dairy milk and select a product with at least 6–10 grams of protein per cup (250 ml). Be sure to choose milks that are fortified with calcium, vitamin D, and vitamin B_{12}. Your best bets are soy milk, pea-based milk, or protein-fortified nut or seed milks. Here are ideas for adding nondairy milks:

   - Pour on hot or cold cereal.
   - Use in pancakes, waffles, and baked goods, such as muffins.
   - Use in smoothies (or other beverages).
   - Use in soups and stews.
   - Add to salad dressings and sauces.
   - Use to make nut creams and puddings, such as Creamy Vanilla Chia Pudding (page 134).

2. **Eat three or more servings of legumes each day.** (1 serving = ½ c./125 ml cooked) Get creative with ways to use beans, lentils, and split peas in meals and snacks:

   - Have a bean burrito for breakfast or experiment with lentil or mung bean pancakes (check out great recipes and videos online).
   - Enjoy bean, lentil, or split pea soup at lunch or dinner. French Canadian Pea Soup (page 152) or Curry in a Hurry (page 154) are delicious choices.
   - Make a sandwich or veggie wrap with hummus or a filling, such as Tangy Chickpea Smash (page 147).
   - Sprinkle sprouted lentils or mung beans on your salad.
   - Add canned beans or a scoop of Full of Beans Salad (page 141) or Lentil Tabouli (page 142) to your green salad.
   - Go for bean-based dinner dishes, such as Easy-Peasy Chili (page 156), Black Bean Stew (page 159), or Stove-Top Baked Beans (page 160).
   - Choose legume-based pastas, such as black bean, chickpea, edamame, or lentil.

3. **Make tofu and tempeh regular features in your diet.** Tofu and tempeh are packed with protein and a good dose of leucine.

- Try some Golden Scrambled Tofu and Veggies (page 129) for breakfast.
- Make a double batch of Tasty Tofu Fingers (pages 132–133) and enjoy with salads, dinner bowls, stir-fries, or straight out of the refrigerator as snacks throughout the day.
- Whip up Rainbow Veggie Fajitas (page 161) or Gado Gado (page 169) for dinner.
- Grill tofu or tempeh or use in stir-fries.
- Add soft tofu to smoothies or puddings.

4. **Add veggie meats.** Veggie versions of burgers, ground round, chicken, beef, or fish are packed with highly digestible protein. Although they are more processed than beans or tofu, they can add variety and protein to a mostly whole-food, plant-based diet. Compare labels for fiber, fat, and sodium content.

   - Try veggie deli slices in sandwiches or on crackers for lunch or snacks.
   - Enjoy a veggie burger or veggie sausage at dinner.
   - Include veggie meat in your stir-fries, stews, chilis, casseroles, or on skewers for a barbecue.
   - Try a veggie meat roast for a special occasion.

5. **Throw on some seeds.** Hemp and pumpkin seeds are often overlooked sources of protein.

   - Eat Gorilla Granola (pages 127–128) for breakfast or put pumpkin or hemp seeds on your cereal.
   - Snack on pumpkin seeds and sunflower seeds or add them to your trail mix.
   - Add hemp seeds to smoothies (such as Green Power Smoothie, page 124), puddings (such as Creamy Vanilla Chia Pudding, page 134), salad dressings (such as Lemon-Tahini Protein-Plus Dressing, page 148), and sauces.
   - Sprinkle seeds on salads and dinner bowls (such as Kale Salad with Orange-Ginger Dressing, page 143, or The Big Bowl, page 164).
   - Use seeds in baked goods, such as Carrot Spice Cookies (page 137).

6. **Feature peanuts and tree nuts in your daily diet.** Peanuts belong to the legume group and therefore are higher in protein, though from a culinary perspective they are used like nuts. Tree nuts can add to total protein intakes.

   - Snack on peanuts and tree nuts.
   - Add peanuts and tree nuts to salads and dinner bowls.
   - Use peanut or tree nut butters on bread instead of margarine or butter.

- Use peanut or tree nut butters in baked goods (such as Double-Chocolate Surprise Cookies, page 135), salad dressings (such as Ginger, Lime, and Miso Dressing, page 150), main dishes (such as Gado Gado, page 169), and smoothies (such as Green Power Smoothie, page 124).

7. **Select higher-protein grains.** In one cup (250 ml) of cooked grains, you get 4–5 grams of protein from rice, 8 grams from quinoa, 10 grams from amaranth or Kamut berries, and 12 grams from spelt berries.

- Use higher-protein grains in breakfast bowls, dinner bowls, and pilafs.
- Sprinkle cooked or sprouted grains on salads.
- Add grains to soups and stews.

8. **Eat your veggies.** While vegetables are not concentrated sources of protein, the amounts can add up. For example, these are the protein contents in various one-cup (250 ml) servings:

- 8 grams for fresh peas.
- More than 5 grams for cooked spinach.
- 4 grams for cooked mushrooms or a medium-size baked potato.
- 3–4 grams for other cooked greens and broccoli.

9. **Feature protein-rich choices at every meal and with some snacks.** When putting together meals and snacks, note the sources of your protein: protein-rich non-dairy milks, beans, lentils, chickpeas, split peas, seeds, nuts, or veggie meats. Add protein boosts to dishes or snacks that typically fall short. When snacking on fruit, add a handful of nuts or seeds, or spread on some nut or seed butter. Add flavored tofu or veggie meats such as pepperoni, ham, or sausage to veggie pizza, and tofu or lentils to lasagna.

10. **Consider adding protein powder.** If you are unable to meet your recommended dietary allowance for protein, you might add some protein powder. (See pages 93–94 for more information.) The people who are most likely to benefit from concentrated protein supplements are strength athletes and seniors.

PROTEIN-PACKED MENUS

W e are providing two sets of menus. The first is an easy menu plan using only a few recipes, while the second uses several of the recipes provided in the next chapter. For each, you will find protein levels suitable for people of different sizes and activity levels (see Key to Sample Menus on page 108). Chapters 2 and 12 provide guidelines for calculating your protein requirements.

Key to Sample Menus

The calculations are based on meeting the recommended dietary allowance (RDA) for protein for adults, teens, and pregnant women as well as expert recommendations for seniors and athletes, plus an additional 10 percent as a safety margin:

Adults—0.9 grams per kilogram of body weight (RDA + 10%)

Teens—0.95 grams per kilogram of body weight (RDA + 10%)

Pregnant women—1.2 grams per kilogram of body weight (RDA + 10%)

Seniors—1.2 grams per kilogram of body weight (expert recommendations + 10%)

Athletes—1.6 grams per kilogram of body weight (expert recommendations + 10%)

TABLE 13.2. Sample menu #1: Fast and easy

MEAL	FOOD	OPTION 1: Total protein in 60 g serving size (G PROTEIN)	OPTION 2: Total protein in 80 g serving size (G PROTEIN)	OPTION 3: Total protein in 100 g serving size (G PROTEIN)	OPTION 4: Total protein in 150 g serving size (G PROTEIN)
Breakfast	Oatmeal or cold cereal	1 c./250 ml (6)	1 c./250 ml (6)	1 c./250 ml (6)	1 c./250 ml (6)
	Soy milk, unsweetened	1 c./250 ml (8)	1 c./250 ml (8)	1 c./250 ml (8)	1 c./250 ml (8)
	Ground flaxseeds	1 T./15 ml (1)	1 T./15 ml (1)	1 T./15 ml (1)	1 T./15 ml (1)
	Strawberries	1 c./250 ml (1)	1 c./250 ml (1)	1 c./250 ml (1)	1 c./250 ml (1)
	Pumpernickel toast	–	1 slice (4)	1 slice (4)	2 slices (8)
	Almond butter	–	1 T./15 ml (4)	1 T./15 ml (4)	2 T./30 ml (8)
Lunch	Whole-grain pita sandwich with hummus, seasoned tofu, and veggies	1 medium pita, ¼ c. hummus, 2 oz. tofu + veg (20)	1 medium pita, ¼ c. hummus, 2 oz. tofu + veg (20)	1 medium pita, ¼ c. hummus, 2 oz. tofu + veg (20)	1 medium pita, ¼ c. hummus, 2 oz. tofu + veg (20)
	Apple	1 medium (1)	1 medium (1)	1 medium (1)	1 medium (1)
	Peanut butter	1 T./15 ml (4)	1 T./15 ml (4)	1 T./15 ml (4)	2 T./30 ml (8)
Dinner	Legume pasta (such as lentil, bean, edamame)	¾ c./185 ml (14)	1 c./250 ml (18)	1¼ c./310 ml (23)	1½ c./375 ml (27)
	Marinara sauce	½ c./125 ml (2)	½ c./125 ml (2)	1 c./250 ml (4)	1 c./250 ml (4)
	Veggie balls	–	–	–	6 (30)
	Green salad with dressing	2 c./500 ml (2)	2 c./500 ml (2)	2 c./500 ml (2)	4 c./1 L (4)
Snacks	Orange	1 (1)	1 (1)	1 (1)	1 (1)
	Trail mix	–	2 oz. (60 g) (8)	1½ oz. (45 g) (6)	2 oz. (60 g) (8)
	Power bar	–	–	1 (15)	1 (15)
TOTAL		60	80	100	150

KEY: T. = tablespoon, c. = cup, oz. = ounce, line — means no amount of the food was consumed. For example, in the 60-gram protein menu, pumpernickel toast, almond butter, trail mix, and the power bar were not consumed.

Sources: US Department of Agriculture (fdc.nal.usda.gov) and ESHA Research (esha.com/products/food-processor).

Total Protein per Day (based on healthy body weight)

Option 1: 60 grams. Suitable for plant-based adults up to 145 pounds (66 kg), teens up to 139 pounds (63 kg), seniors up to 110 pounds (50 kg), and pregnant women whose pre-pregnancy weight is up to 110 pounds (50 kg).

Option 2: 80 grams. Suitable for plant-based adults up to 194 pounds (88 kg), teens up to 185 pounds (84 kg), seniors up to 147 pounds (67 kg), pregnant women whose pre-pregnancy weight is up to 147 pounds (67 kg), and athletes up to 110 pounds (50 kg).

Option 3: 100 grams. Suitable for plant-based adults up to 244 pounds (111 kg), teens up to 231 pounds (105 kg), seniors up to 183 pounds (83 kg), pregnant women whose pre-pregnancy weight is up to 183 pounds (83 kg), and athletes up to 139 pounds (63 kg).

Option 4: 150 grams. Suitable for plant-based athletes up to 207 pounds (94 kg).

TABLE 13.3. Sample Menu #2: Protein plus

MEAL	FOOD	OPTION 1: Total protein in 60 g serving size (G PROTEIN)	OPTION 2: Total protein in 80 g serving size (G PROTEIN)	OPTION 3: Total protein in 100 g serving size (G PROTEIN)	OPTION 4: Total protein in 140 g serving size (G PROTEIN)
Breakfast	Powered-Up Overnight Oats (page 125)	1¼ c./310 ml (13)	1¼ c./310 ml (13)	½ recipe (20)	½ recipe (20)
	Soy milk, unsweetened	½ c./125 ml (4)	½ c./125 ml (4)	¾ c./185 ml (6)	1 c./250 ml (8)
	Blueberries	1 c./250 ml (1)	1 c./250 ml (1)	1 c./250 ml (1)	1 c./250 ml (1)
Lunch	Power Greens Salad (page 138)	4 c./1 L (3)	4 c./1 L (3)	4 c./1 L (3)	4 c./1 L (3)
	Baked tofu (page 132)	2 oz./60 g (9)	4 oz./120 g (18)	4 oz./120 g (18)	4 oz./120 g (18)
	Chickpeas	–	–	–	1 c./250 ml (8)
	Quinoa	½ c./125 ml (4)	½ c./125 ml (4)	½ c./125 ml (4)	1 c./250 ml (8)
	Extra veggies (sugar snap peas, avocado, carrots, broccoli)	1 c./250 ml (2)	1 c./250 ml (2)	1 c./250 ml (2)	1½ c./375 ml (3)
	Lemon-Tahini Protein-Plus Dressing (page 148)	2 T./30 ml (4)	3 T./45 ml (6)	3 T./45 ml (6)	⅓ c./85 ml (9)
Dinner	Easy-Peasy Chili (page 156)	1 c./250 ml (14)	1½ c./375 ml (20)	2 c./375 ml (27)	2 c./500 ml (27)
	Kale Salad with Orange-Ginger Dressing (page 143)	1 c./250 ml (6)	1 c./250 ml (6)	1 c./250 ml (6)	2 c./500 ml (11)
Snacks	Double-Chocolate Surprise Cookies (page 135)	–	–	2 (7)	2 (7)
	Green Power Smoothie (page 124)	–	–	–	1 recipe (3 c./750 ml) (24)
	Mango	–	1 medium (3)	–	1 medium (3)
TOTAL		60	80	100	150

KEY: T. = tablespoon, c. = cup, oz. = ounce, line – means no amount of the food was consumed.

Sources: US Department of Agriculture (fdc.nal.usda.gov) and ESHA Research (esha.com/products/food-processor).

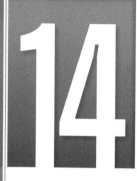

The Protein-Powered Kitchen

N ow that you are well versed in the facts and fallacies that surround plant protein and its impressive benefits, let's turn our attention to the kitchen! In this chapter we offer some basic cooking guidelines, and in chapter 15 you'll discover 30 delicious protein-packed, plant-based recipes divided into three categories:

1. Breakfast and On-the-Go Recipes
2. Salads and Dressings
3. Hearty Soups and Mains

These recipes are loaded with healthful ingredients and are simple to prepare. We provide a nutritional analysis with each recipe. The analysis is based on metric measures of ingredients, without optional ingredients or as we have specified in individual recipes. If there is a series of choices (such as types of greens), the analysis will be based on the first choice listed.

GET COMFY IN THE KITCHEN

I f you are just learning to cook from scratch, this preface will help kick-start your culinary adventure. Even if you have had decades of experience in the kitchen, some techniques employed in healthful, plant-based cuisine may be new to you. Be sure to check out the special sections "Cooking Beans" (pages 119–120) and "Cooking Grains" (pages 120–122). These handy guides will be go-to references throughout your plant-based cooking experience.

To save time and frustration, before you dive into the recipes, do a kitchen audit and make any necessary adjustments:

Gather essential pieces of kitchen equipment. These are baking dishes, baking sheets, a can opener, a chef's knife, a colander, cookware (such as pots, pans, and skillets in various sizes), a cutting board, a ladle, measuring cups and spoons, mixing bowls, parchment paper or silicone baking mats, a paring knife, a peeler, rubber spatulas, a steamer basket, tongs, a turner (that is, a flipper or metal spatula), a whisk, and wooden spoons. Consider investing in a heavy-duty high-powered blender and a food processor. These appliances will help you prepare dressings, spreads, sauces, and puddings in a jiffy. Also consider purchasing a multipurpose programmable pressure cooker to make cooking beans and grains a breeze.

Determine your best ways of acquiring healthful plant-based foods in your area. You may find local farmers' markets, organic delivery services, co-ops, bulk stores, ethnic stores, and natural food stores that you can frequent. You may decide to plant a garden or grow sprouts or herbs at home. For items that are hard to source locally, check online. Stock your pantry well so you are set up for food prep.

Consider taking a plant-based cooking class. Explore the possibilities both locally and online. A cooking school specializing in plant-based whole foods will familiarize you with ingredients, recipes, and flavor combinations to help you replace your favorite comfort foods as well as broaden your culinary horizons. Look online for a range of engaging courses.

Find resources that keep your creative juices flowing. Cookbooks, magazines, websites, and videos can inspire and motivate you to try new things. Embrace the adventure.

Surround yourself with other plant-based eaters. Look for groups, meetups, and events in your area. If resources are few and far between, find support online.

THE PLANT-BASED PANTRY

If you are shifting from an omnivorous diet to a healthy, sustainable, plant-based diet, you may be in the market for a pantry makeover. Of course, you'll want to clean out the refrigerator and freezer as well. Having an organized kitchen will help support your transition to a healthier lifestyle. It also creates a more efficient and enjoyable experience in the kitchen. Following are four simple steps to guide you through this process.

Step 1: Take stock of what is currently in your pantry. Set aside the foods that are keepers based on your commitment to plant-based eating and to your health.

Step 2: Give away or dispose of foods that no longer serve you. These include items that are not plant-based and items that fall below your standards for nutrition.

Step 3: Organize your pantry, refrigerator, and freezer. Make room for lidded mason jars and other airtight containers so you can store grains and beans in the pantry and nuts, seeds, and leftovers in the refrigerator or freezer. Labeling the containers makes finding and accessing these items a breeze.

Step 4: Stock up on essential provisions. Start by purchasing staples and ingredients that are specific to the recipes you are planning to make. Dry ingredients can be purchased in appropriate amounts and stored in sealed containers in a cool, dry place. Most are best used within a year, although many will last longer. For the best prices, look for sources that offer grains and legumes in bulk. Ethnic stores and the ethnic sections of supermarkets and natural food stores are often good places to find legumes or unfamiliar ingredients at reasonable prices. Here are some tips for each category of food:

Whole grains. Start with four or five common grains, such as barley, old-fashioned rolled oats, quinoa, and black, brown, or red rice. When you have mastered the preparation of a few common grains, try a few others, such as farro, Kamut, and wild rice. You may also keep some heavy whole-grain bread, tortillas, and pasta on hand. Store bread you will not use in two or three days in the freezer.

Legumes. Legumes are the key to a protein-rich pantry. Include a variety of dried or canned beans, split peas, and lentils. As you begin stocking your plant-based pantry, include one or two types of lentils (such as black, brown, French, green, or red), some split peas, and three or four types of beans (such as black beans, chickpeas, great northern beans, kidney beans, navy beans, or pinto beans). Add a legume-based pasta made from legumes like black beans, chickpeas, edamame, or lentils. These pasta varieties provide about triple the protein of grain-based alternatives. Stock your refrigerator with hummus, tempeh, tofu, and veggie burgers or sausages. Have a bag of edamame in the freezer, as well as your favorite veggie meats. While veggie burgers, sausages, and other veggie meats are not necessary, they are concentrated sources of highly digestible protein, and they can add variety to your menus. However, they are often very processed and high in sodium, so compare labels and keep your intake moderate.

Nuts and seeds. Nuts and seeds are treasured plant-based staples. The most popular nuts include almonds, Brazil nuts, cashews, hazelnuts, pecans, and walnuts. Ensure you have raw cashews on hand, because they serve as the base of many sauces and dressings. Peanuts, while technically a legume, tend to be included in this category because, from a culinary perspective, they are used as nuts. Seeds are even more concentrated in protein than most nuts. Include the excellent sources of omega-3 fatty acids—chia seeds, ground flaxseeds, and hemp seeds. For zinc and other minerals, add pumpkin, sesame, and sunflower seeds to your list of essentials. Store shelled nuts and seeds in the refrigerator or freezer; keep out only enough to use within a week or two. Finally, keep one or two nut (e.g., almond or cashew) or seed butters (e.g., tahini or sunflower butter) on hand.

Vegetables. Buy fresh produce as you need it and buy it in season. It's preferable to choose organic and locally grown produce. Purchase what you can use within a week, with the exception of winter squashes and most root vegetables, which can last for weeks and even months when they are stored in a cool, dry place. For convenience, you can buy frozen vegetables, such as peas and corn. Canned vegetables tend to be more heavily processed and higher in sodium than frozen vegetables, so choose them less often and check labels. Include jarred or canned tomato sauce, diced tomatoes, and tomato paste. Make sure to keep enough leafy greens on hand that you can eat them at least once a day. A fun goal when selecting vegetables is to include something from every color of the rainbow. Here are some examples:

- Green: asparagus, basil, bok choy, broccoli, broccolini, Brussels sprouts, cabbage, celery, cilantro, collard greens, cucumbers, green beans, green onions, green peppers, kale, lettuces, napa cabbage, parsley, spinach, sprouts, zucchini
- Pink-red: beets, peppers, radishes, tomatoes
- Purple-blue: eggplant, purple asparagus, purple carrots, purple cauliflower, purple potatoes, red cabbage
- White-beige: cauliflower, daikon, garlic, kohlrabi, onions, potatoes
- Yellow-orange: carrots, corn, peppers, golden beets, squash, sweet potatoes

Fruits. Fruits are another important staple. Like vegetables, it's best to purchase fruits that are in season. Stock your kitchen with a wide variety of fruit—try citrus fruits (such as grapefruit, lemons, limes, and oranges), berries, melons, and other in-season fruit such as apples, apricots, bananas, grapes, kiwi, peaches, pears, and plums. Dried fruits—such as apricots, cherries, dates (medjool and the more common deglet noor), figs, peaches, pears, prunes, and raisins—serve as ideal sweeteners for treats, so include at least two or three varieties in your pantry.

Plant-based nondairy products. Nondairy milks, cheeses, yogurts, and other dairy replacements are widely available in supermarkets. Choose milks that are unsweetened and fortified (that is, enriched). Soy and pea milks stand out for their protein content. Vegan cheeses vary wildly in their nutritional value —some are predominantly oils and starches (these are the less nutritious choices), while those based on cultured nuts or seeds are far more healthful options. Read the labels of nondairy yogurt and ice cream products, because many of these contain as much added sugar as their dairy counterparts.

Herbs and spices. The sky's the limit when it comes to herbs and spices. Your choices will vary with your cultural traditions, taste preferences, and kitchen space. Some basics are allspice, basil, bay leaves, cayenne, chili powder, cinnamon, cumin, curry powder, dill, garlic powder (or garlic granules), ginger, marjoram, mint, nutmeg, onion powder (or onion flakes), oregano, paprika, pepper, rosemary, sage, salt, savory, thyme, and turmeric. Seasoning blends are also a great addition to enliven an entire dish. If you have the space, grow fresh herbs (even in pots on your balcony); this is an economical way to add flavor to your meals. If it's feasible, purchase herbs and spices from a reputable spice shop or opt for organic products.

Other ingredients. You will need some cornstarch, dark chocolate chips or chunks, unsweetened cocoa powder, unsweetened shredded dried coconut, and vanilla (in the form of whole pods, powder, or extract). You will also possibly need a couple of sweeteners, such as natural maple syrup and organic blackstrap molasses. Keep handy a few condiments, such as Bragg Liquid Aminos, coconut aminos, soy sauce, or tamari; hot sauce; miso; mustards; nutritional yeast flakes; olives; pickles; vegetable broth; vinegars (such as apple cider, balsamic, rice, and wine vinegars); and a small amount of high-quality vegetable oil—such as avocado, olive, or sesame—or a high-quality spray oil.

THE LOWDOWN ON ADDED SUGAR, OIL, AND SALT

In the plant-based community, there are diverse opinions about the use of added salt, oil, and sugar. Some people follow a diet that excludes added sugar, oil, and salt, while others use these flavor enhancers quite liberally. From a culinary perspective, these items can add a lot of flavor, even with judicious use. From a nutritional perspective, they are generally unnecessary and potentially damaging to health, particularly when used in excess. It makes sense to minimize the use of these ingredients, especially for those who have or are at risk for chronic diseases such as heart disease or type 2 diabetes. On the other hand, there is little evidence to suggest that using small amounts is harmful. You can easily adjust the recipes in this book to suit your palate and your unique health goals. Let's explore each of these additions in a little more detail and discover ways they can be replaced with whole foods.

Added Sugar

Health authorities recommend keeping a lid on added sugar. Guidelines in North America and many European countries recommend limiting added sugar to not more than 10 percent of a person's total calories. The World Health Organization has the same upper limit but adds that a further reduction to not more than 5 percent of calories would provide greater health benefits. In a typical 2,000-calorie diet, 10 percent of those calories would be 12 teaspoons (60 ml) of sugar per day and 5 percent of those calories would be 6 teaspoons (30 ml) of sugar per day. Note that 1 teaspoon (5 ml) of sugar is equal to about 4 grams of sugar on a food label. While this may seem like a lot of sugar, you might be surprised how much sugar commonly consumed foods contain. For example, a 16-ounce cola contains about 12 teaspoons (60 ml) of sugar; a large cinnamon bun has about 10 teaspoons (50 ml); and 1 cup (250 ml) of frozen yogurt contains about 8 teaspoons (40 ml). It is easy to exceed the upper limits when we adhere to a standard Western diet.

Fortunately, there are a lot of great ways to decrease your sugar intake:

- Drink water instead of sugary beverages.
- Use fresh or dried fruits to replace sugar in salad dressings, baked goods, and other treats.
- Add seasonings, such as vanilla extract and ground cinnamon.
- Use fresh fruit to satisfy your sweet tooth.
- Cut sugar in half in traditional recipes and select more nutrient-dense sweeteners, such as organic blackstrap molasses or natural maple syrup.

Added Oil

In most cuisines, foods are commonly sautéed in oil. While many healthy populations use some oil in their cooking, there are three key reasons to limit your intake. First, oil has a lot of calories (120 calories per 1 tablespoon/15 ml) and very few nutrients. Second, when oils are heated to high temperatures, they tend to produce products of oxidation that have negative effects on health. Third, many popular oils (such as corn, grapeseed, safflower, and sunflower oils) are very high in omega-6 fatty acids, which can interfere with the body's metabolism of omega-3 fatty acids, especially when they are a regular feature of the diet.

Here are tips to minimize your use of added oil:

- Try your hand at dry sautéing. Surprisingly, dry sautéing is actually the preferred method of browning for high-moisture vegetables like mushrooms. It also works well for onions. Using low or medium-low heat and high-quality heavy cookware with a lid helps prevent sticking. Cook onions, stirring frequently, until they have caramelized.
- Use vegetable broth, water, or nonalcoholic wine instead of oil for sautéing.

- In baked goods, use nut or seed butters in place of oil. Or try applesauce, mashed bananas, or prune purée. Decrease the amount of other sweeteners if replacing oil with fruit.
- In salad dressings, use avocados, nuts, seeds, or their butters in place of oil.
- If using oils in salad dressings, select those that are rich in omega-3 fatty acids—such as flax or hemp seed oil—and keep quantities small.
- If using oil as a flavoring (such as toasted sesame oil in a peanut sauce), include the smallest amount possible.
- Avoid deep-fried foods and limit processed foods high in added oils.

Added Salt

Sodium is an essential nutrient, and the minimum physiological requirement is 500 milligrams per day (the amount in one-fifth of a teaspoon of salt). Endurance athletes and those who are working in the sun have higher requirements as sodium is lost in perspiration.

However, too much salt can increase the risk of hypertension and cardiovascular disease. To decrease that risk, some health advocates suggest eliminating added salt altogether, as many foods provide small amounts of sodium. In North America, the National Academy of Sciences has set an upper limit for sodium called the Chronic Disease Risk Reduction Intake (CDRR). Sodium intake above this limit is associated with increased risk to one's health. For adults, the CDRR suggests reducing sodium intakes if they exceed 2,300 milligrams per day (the limits are lower for those under 14 years of age). The American Heart Association suggests an ideal intake of no more than 1,500 milligrams per day. This is an excellent target for those with high blood pressure or cardiovascular disease. However, athletes who sweat a lot during training require more sodium. American adults average more than 3,400 milligrams of sodium per day, with over 70 percent coming from processed foods.

Most experienced cooks know that nothing heightens the flavor of food like salt—even a small amount can work wonders. Many recipes will instruct cooks to "season with salt to taste" because the amount of salt needed to hit the sweet spot will depend on the quality of your ingredients, your palate, and the type of salt used. Old-fashioned iodized salt is a reasonable choice, especially if you are relying on salt as a primary source of iodine. It is versatile and inexpensive, and it dissolves quickly. Kosher salt has larger crystals and is less dense. One teaspoon (5 ml) of kosher salt has about the same amount of sodium as about one-half to two-thirds of a teaspoon (2–3 ml) of table salt. When adding salt to a recipe, use just a little, as it is easy to add more, but an oversalted dish is not so easy to fix.

Here are tips to decrease your sodium intake:

- Decrease salt in recipes or omit salt altogether.
- Add a squeeze of lemon or lime or a splash of vinegar to enhance flavor.
- Add extra garlic, herbs, onion, and spices.
- Use fresh herbs instead of dried.
- Add some nutritional yeast flakes to the dish.
- Be very selective with condiments and processed foods.
- Read and compare food labels. There are often significant differences in the sodium content of canned tomatoes, crackers, sauces, soups, and even peanut butter.
- Use salt-free or lower-sodium options, such as low-sodium tamari and unsalted vegetable broth.

GETTING RECIPES RIGHT

Most people have experienced a recipe disaster at one time or another. These six simple steps will help you make the most of every recipe you try:

1. **Read the recipe from start to finish before you begin.** Reading a recipe through once or twice before you start will help ensure that you have all the necessary ingredients and tools, have done any required advance preparation, and have set aside sufficient time to cook.

2. **Prep your ingredients.** Gather all the ingredients listed, then chop, dice, mince, or complete any other type of preparation that the recipe calls for. Arrange your ingredients on a cutting board or in bowls. If a recipe calls for something that takes a long time to cook (such as cooked grains or beans), prepare those ahead of time.

3. **Measure ingredients carefully.** When you measure carefully, your chances of success are greatly enhanced, especially when it comes to baking. Inaccurate measurements can lead to dishes that are too dry, wet, spicy, or bland.

4. **Make food selections carefully.** A dish will only be as good as the ingredients used to make it. Fresh ingredients that are in season or from your garden or local farmers' market are almost always your best bet. The flavors of fresh herbs and freshly squeezed citrus juice are outstanding, and fresh garlic and ginger taste richer than their dried counterparts.

5. **Be savvy with substitutions.** You can make substitutions in recipes, but it is generally a good idea to make a recipe as directed the first time you try it. Some swaps are simple, such as replacing navy beans with a slightly larger variety of white beans (like great northern beans), tofu with tempeh, or cooked rice with cooked quinoa. You can replace vegetables and fruits to suit

your taste and what you have on hand. However, be careful to make the replacements reasonable. You would not replace tomatoes in a tomato-based sauce, but you could add herbs, such as basil or oregano, to suit your palate. As your culinary skills improve, you will feel more comfortable making substitutions.

6. **Set up your counter space.** Arrange and organize your ingredients and equipment according to which items you'll use first. If your counter space is limited, consider bringing a small portable table or island on wheels into the kitchen when you need additional surface area.

KITCHEN WIZARDRY

Making the switch to cooking with whole, plant-based foods may feel a little overwhelming. It can mean more time in the kitchen when compared to cooking according to standard Western diets, especially while you adjust to new recipes. However, after you have found some favorite recipes, the process becomes simpler. Think of it as an investment in your health and the health of your family. Make meal preparation a priority and allow sufficient time, so that you can enjoy the process. Of course, life gets crazy at times, so it is nice to know that there are ways to lighten your load. Here are our top five plant-based kitchen shortcuts:

1. **Cook in batches.** Once a week (or more often if needed), cook a pot of beans and a pot of grains, and prepare a giant undressed salad of leafy greens (without cucumbers or tomatoes, which can be added before serving). Prepare a favorite dressing, bake granola, and bake potatoes, squash, or sweet potatoes while the oven is hot. Blend a chia pudding. With these staples ready to go, putting together a meal will be a snap. A breakfast bowl could include fresh or stewed fruit; grains; granola; and chia seeds, ground flaxseeds, or hemp seeds (or a mixture). An undressed salad could serve as a foundation for lunch with the addition of grains, beans, steamed sweet squash, and salad dressing. Dinner could be a bowl of grains, steamed vegetables, beans, nuts or seeds, and dressing.

2. **Double or triple recipes.** Buy single-portion containers that can be frozen and heated or microwaved. When you discover favorite soups and main course recipes, make enough to freeze leftovers for quick meals. This is especially helpful for labor-intensive dishes, such as baked goods, lasagna, loaves, and veggie patties.

3. **Soak beans and grains for faster cooking.** Presoaking beans and grains can cut cooking time by up to 50 percent, improve digestibility, and limit antinutrients that hinder mineral absorption. Ideally, soak beans and grains for 8–12 hours. Larger grains and legumes will take longer than smaller ones.

4. **Prep veggies.** Prepping some of your veggies for instant consumption can save time and will likely improve your intake. Many vegetables can be washed, cut, and stored in airtight containers for use within a day or two—this method works well for broccoli, cauliflower, celery, peppers, and other veggies that do not easily discolor or wilt. It is best not to cut avocados, cucumbers, and tomatoes too far in advance, as doing so hastens their demise. Greens and sprouts can be carefully rinsed and put in covered containers for quick use in dinner bowls and smoothies. When you get home from the market (or when your bin arrives on your doorstep), immediately prepare a giant salad that will last, refrigerated, for a few days (see page 138). It helps to have a large bowl with a lid for this purpose.

5. **Organize your kitchen equipment for ease of use.** Keep your blender, food processor, and electric pressure cooker within easy reach. Arrange knives and other kitchen tools so you can access them quickly. When tools are handy, you'll be more apt to use them.

COOKING BEANS

Cooking dried beans, peas, and lentils is easy, practical, and economical. Dried legumes can be stored for a year or longer in a cool, dry place. Generally, it is best to use them within a year of purchase, as the older they get, the drier they will become and the longer they will need to cook to become tender. (Note that canned beans are also good sources of minerals and protein.)

When cooking legumes, make enough so you can freeze some. Put them in a freezer bag or labeled container; you can store them in the freezer for six months. Cooking large quantities of legumes at one time allows you to have several different types ready whenever you need them.

Dried beans, peas, and lentils should be rinsed before cooking. Also look through them carefully and remove any small stones, pieces of debris, and shriveled or discolored beans. It is best to presoak most beans prior to cooking, as this will help remove oligosaccharides and improve the legumes' digestibility and nutrient availability. Split peas, lentils, and mung beans do not require presoaking, although a short soak (2–4 hours) may improve their digestibility.

Here are basic guidelines for the preparation of dried beans:

1. **Soak the beans.** Presoaking beans decreases their cooking time, mitigates the oligosaccharides responsible for flatulence, and improves their digestibility. There are two main ways to soak beans: the traditional soak and the quick soak.
   a. **The traditional soak.** Put the beans in a large bowl or saucepan and add 5 cups (1.25 L) of water per 1 cup (250 ml) of beans. Soak for 8–12 hours.

It is acceptable to soak beans for up to 24 hours but be sure to put them in the fridge if soaking for more than 12 hours. Soaking for more than 24 hours can negatively affect the texture and flavor of the beans. Drain the beans and discard the soaking water. Rinse the beans with cold water before cooking them.

b. **The quick soak.** Put the beans in a large saucepan and add 4 cups (1 L) of water for every 1 cup (250 ml) of beans. Bring to a boil over high heat and boil for 2–3 minutes. Remove the saucepan from the heat, cover, and let stand for at least 1 hour. Drain and rinse the beans prior to cooking them.

2. **Cook the drained, presoaked beans.** If you are using a multipurpose cooker or another type of cooker, follow the instructions provided by the manufacturer. If using the stove top, put the beans in a large saucepan and add 3 cups (750 ml) of water per 1 cup (250 ml) of dried beans. Bring to a boil over high heat, decrease the heat to medium-low, and simmer gently until the beans are tender, 1–2 hours. Generally speaking, the larger or older the beans, the longer the cooking time. Since beans expand during cooking, add warm water as needed to ensure they are always covered. Skim off any foam that rises to the top, as this contains oligosaccharides that can cause flatulence. Beans are done when you can mash them on the roof of your mouth with your tongue.

If you'd like to flavor the legumes while they cook, add acidic ingredients (such as vinegar, tomatoes, or citrus juice) near the end of the cooking time, when the beans are tender. If these ingredients are added sooner, they can make the beans tough and slow the cooking process. Herbs and spices (including salt) can be added at the beginning of the cooking process, if desired.

Split peas, lentils, and mung beans do not require presoaking and need less time to cook. Split peas take 45–60 minutes, lentils take 30–45 minutes, and red lentils can be cooked in 15–20 minutes.

COOKING GRAINS

Intact whole grains are cooked using the same methods as brown rice and quinoa, though amounts of water and cooking times vary. Rinse the grains before cooking them to remove dirt and debris. Bring the water to a boil in a heavy saucepan with a tight-fitting lid. Add the grains, return to a boil, then lower the heat, cover, and simmer until the grains are tender. The chart that follows provides details about the amount of water needed and cooking times. Using vegetable broth in place of water or adding a pinch of salt to the water will provide a flavor boost. In general, larger grains need more water and a longer cooking time. The time needed will also vary depending on the saucepan and the stove you are using. Grains are done when they are tender, so if they are not sufficiently tender when the time is up, add more water and continue cooking. You can cut cooking time in half by presoaking grains in the allotted amount of water for 4–12 hours. Then cook them in the soaking water or in fresh water. Many whole grains will fluff up if you turn off the heat and leave them covered for about 5 minutes after all the water has been absorbed. This will also help the grains separate and not stick together as much when they are stored. If the cooked grains are stuck to the bottom of the saucepan, turn off the heat, add a small amount of liquid, cover the saucepan, and let it sit for about 10 minutes. The grains will loosen, making them easier to serve; this technique will make cleaning the saucepan easier as well.

When cooking grains, make enough to last for several days. Add cooked whole grains to breakfast or dinner bowls, soups, salads, and main dishes. You can freeze individual or meal-size portions of cooked grains in labeled containers for six months.

Electric Pressure-Cooking

A wonderful addition to any plant-based kitchen is a programmable electric pressure cooker. This handy appliance cuts cooking time considerably. Plus, it frees you to be elsewhere than in the kitchen! It works beautifully for cooking both beans and grains. Here are some of the perks of an electric pressure cooker:

- It is super energy efficient. The cooking chamber is insulated, and the amount of liquid required for cooking is much less than with traditional cooking methods.

- It retains a food's nutrients, minimizing nutritional losses.

- It preserves a food's appearance. Cooking in open containers, which exposes food to oxygen, can lead to color loss in food. Pressure-cooking uses steam, allowing for the retention of the food's bright colors. It also helps retain shape in beans, because they cook evenly and tend not to split, break, or fall apart.

- It heightens flavor. Because beans are cooked using less liquid, they retain flavor.

- It eliminates potential bacterial contamination. Pressure-cooking allows water to boil at temperatures that exceed 212 degrees F (100 degrees C), destroying harmful bacteria.

TABLE 14.1. Grain cooking times and yields

GRAIN	COOKING TIME (MINUTES)	YIELD
1 cup (250 ml) grains plus 2 cups (500 ml) water		
Amaranth	15–20	2½ cups/625 ml
Buckwheat	20	4 cups/1 L
Bulgur	10–12	3 cups/750 ml
Quinoa	12–15	3 cups/750 ml
1 cup (250 ml) grains plus 2½ cups (625 ml) water		
Brown rice	30–45	3 cups/750 ml
Farro	25–40	3 cups/750 ml
Millet	25–35	4 cups/1 L
1 cup (250 ml) grains plus 3 cups (750 ml) water		
Barley	45–60	3½ cups/875 ml
Teff	20	2½ cups/625 ml
Wild rice	45–55	3½ cups/875 ml
1 cup (250 ml) grains plus 4 cups (1 L) water		
Kamut, spelt, or rye berries	Soak for 8–12 hours* + 45–60	3 cups/750 ml
Oats, steel-cut or groats	30	3 cups/750 ml
Sorghum	25–40	3 cups/750 ml
Wheat berries	Soak for 8–12 hours* + 45–60	2½ cups/625 ml

*Soaking is optional, but the cooking time will increase to 75–90 minutes without soaking.
Source: wholegrainscouncil.org/recipes/cooking-whole-grains.

References for this chapter are online at https://plant-poweredprotein.com/references.

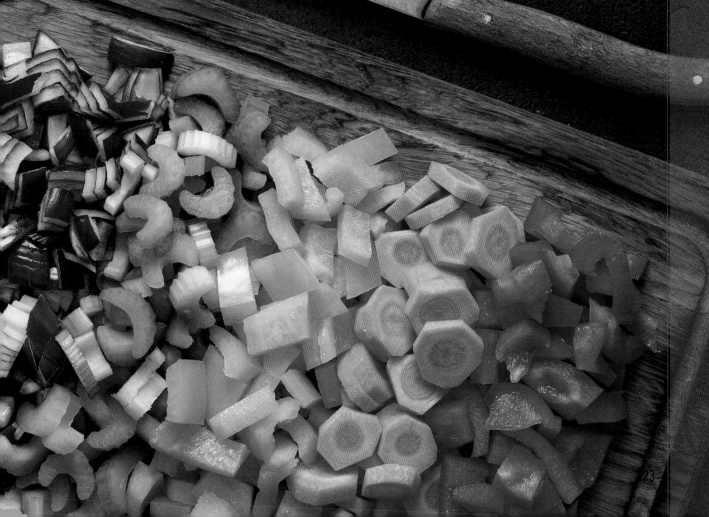

23

GREEN Power Smoothie

Smoothies are popular for breakfast and snacks because they are quick and easy to make, nutrient-dense, and super portable. Including frozen ingredients is the key to extra-thick smoothies.

3 cups (750 ml) kale or other green, packed

1½ cups (375 ml) fortified unsweetened soy milk or other nondairy milk

1 frozen or fresh banana

½ cup (125 ml) frozen or fresh pineapple, mango, or strawberries

3 tablespoons (45 ml) hemp seeds

Put the kale, milk, banana, pineapple, and hemp seeds in a blender and process until smooth. Serve. This smoothie keeps for 1 day in the refrigerator.

Add the boosters at the same time as the other ingredients and process until smooth.

OPTIONAL PROTEIN BOOSTERS (or check labels for protein content)

- ¾ cup (185 ml) frozen peas: adds 5 grams of protein
- 5 ounces (150 g) soft tofu: adds 12 grams of protein
- 1 scoop vegan protein powder: adds 10–15 grams of protein
- 2 tablespoons (30 ml) peanut butter: adds 8 grams of protein

OPTIONAL VEGGIE BOOSTERS

- 1 cup (250 ml) sliced cucumber
- ½ cup (125 ml) sunflower sprouts
- 1 small carrot
- 1 stalk celery

NUTRITION NOTES: The basic recipe with soy milk provides 24 grams of protein for the whole recipe; choosing a fortified milk will increase your intake of calcium and vitamins D and B_{12}. The optional protein boosters will further amp up protein. The optional veggie boosters will add antioxidants and protective phytochemicals.

Per recipe (750 ml) without boosters:

Calories: 508

Protein: 24 g

Leucine: 1,934 mg

Fat: 21 g

Carbohydrate: 64 g

Fiber: 8 g

Minerals:

Iron: 5.3 mg

Zinc: 4.6 mg

Calcium: 590 mg

Sodium: 205 mg

Percent of calories from:

Protein 17%

Fat 36%

Carbohydrate 47%

POWERED-UP Overnight Oats

This nourishing breakfast is prepared the night before for an almost instant meal. Soaking enhances the digestibility of the grains and increases mineral absorption. Replace some of the milk with nondairy yogurt for a traditional European twist.

1 cup (250 ml) old-fashioned rolled oats or steel-cut oats

3 tablespoons (45 ml) hemp seeds

2 tablespoons (30 ml) chopped almonds or other nuts

2 tablespoons (30 ml) raisins or other dried fruit

1 tablespoon (15 ml) chia seeds

¼ teaspoon (1 ml) ground cinnamon

1¼ cups (310 ml) fortified unsweetened soy milk or other nondairy milk

2 cups (500 ml) sliced or chopped fresh fruit or berries (such as apples, apricots, bananas, blackberries, blueberries, mangoes, peaches, pears, raspberries, or strawberries)

Put the oats, hemp seeds, almonds, raisins, chia seeds, cinnamon, and milk in a large bowl and stir to combine. Cover and refrigerate for 8–12 hours. Stir in the fresh fruit just before serving. Stored in a sealed container in the refrigerator, the oats (without the fresh fruit) will keep for 2 days.

SERVING SUGGESTION: Serve with fortified nondairy milk. Sprinkle with Gorilla Granola (page 127) for crunch.

TIP: If you will be enjoying this recipe on the go, prepare it in a mason jar.

Per one-half recipe (463 ml):

Calories: 596

Protein: 20 g

Leucine: 1,562 mg

Fat: 20 g

Carbohydrate: 92 g

Fiber: 13 g

Minerals:

Iron: 5.3 mg

Zinc: 2.6 mg

Calcium: 297 mg

Sodium: 63 mg

Percent of calories from:

Protein 13%

Fat 29%

Carbohydrate 58%

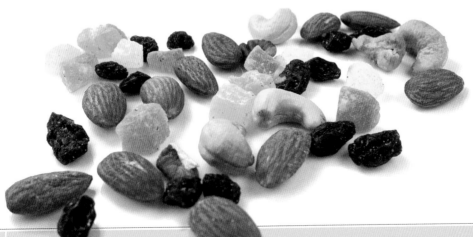

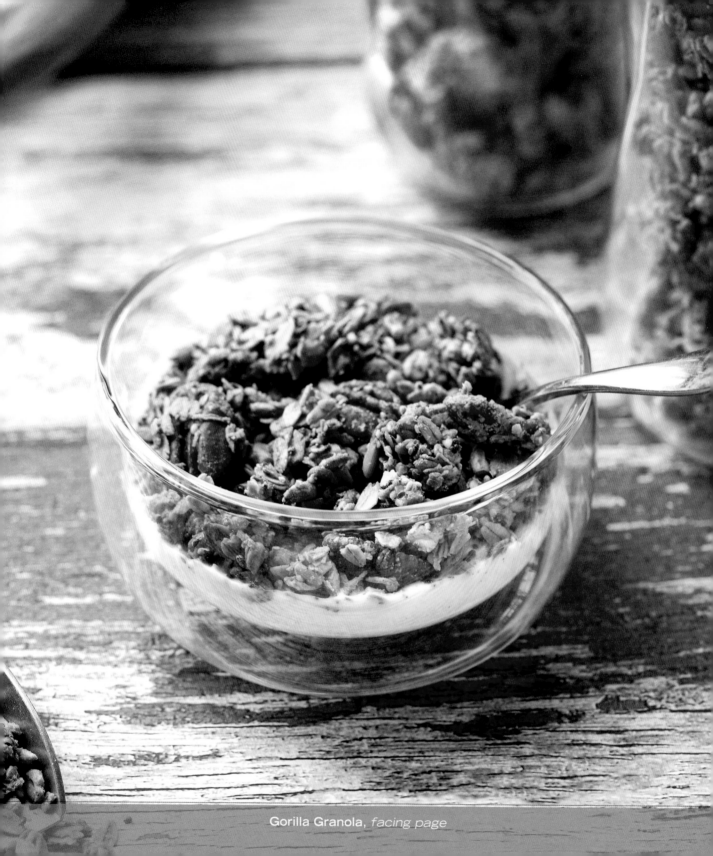

Gorilla Granola, *facing page*

Gorilla Granola WITH TWO OPTIONS

This granola is loaded with nuts, seeds, and nut or seed butter, which gives it a protein edge compared to traditional granola. It can be enjoyed on its own as a snack, with fruit and milk for breakfast, or as a topping for muesli, breakfast bowls, puddings, or frozen fruit ice cream. There are two ways to prepare this recipe: Option 1 is made with whole foods, and Option 2 is a slightly sweeter version using natural maple syrup.

OPTION 1: WHOLE-FOODS GRANOLA

WET INGREDIENTS

1 small seedless orange, peeled and coarsely chopped

1 small banana, broken into chunks

½ cup (125 ml) pitted soft dates, packed

⅓ cup (85 ml) nut or seed butter

2 teaspoons (10 ml) ground cinnamon

1 teaspoon (5 ml) vanilla extract

OPTION 2: MAPLE-NUT GRANOLA

WET INGREDIENTS

½ cup (125 ml) nut or seed butter

⅓ cup (85 ml) natural maple syrup

2 teaspoons (10 ml) ground cinnamon

1 teaspoon (5 ml) vanilla extract

OPTION 1: Put the orange, banana, dates, nut butter, cinnamon, and vanilla extract in a blender. Process, starting on low speed and gradually increasing the speed, until smooth.

OPTION 2: Put the nut butter, maple syrup, cinnamon, and vanilla extract in a large bowl. Stir vigorously until smooth.

Recipe continues on the following page.

Per 1 cup (250 ml)*:
Calories: 549
Protein: 20 g
Leucine: 1,701 mg
Fat: 38 g
Carbohydrate: 42 g
Fiber: 13 g

Minerals:
Iron: 5.3 mg
Zinc: 3.9 mg
Calcium: 168 mg
Sodium: 27 mg

Percent of calories from:
Protein 14%
Fat 58%
Carbohydrate 28%

*Based on Option 1
(with almond butter)

OPTIONS 1 AND 2

DRY INGREDIENTS

3 cups (750 ml) old-fashioned rolled oats

1½ cups (375 ml) raw sunflower seeds

1 cup (250 ml) whole or coarsely chopped raw nuts (such as almonds, cashews, or pecans)

¾ cup (185 ml) raw pumpkin seeds

½ cup (125 ml) hemp seeds

½ cup (125 ml) chia seeds

½ cup (125 ml) unsweetened shredded dried coconut

½ cup (125 ml) currants or raisins (optional)

Preheat the oven to 275 degrees F (135 degrees C). Line 2 large baking pans with silicone mats or parchment paper or mist with cooking spray.

Put the oats, sunflower seeds, nuts, pumpkin seeds, hemp seeds, chia seeds, and coconut in a large bowl. Add the wet ingredients for either Option 1 or Option 2 and stir or mix with your hands until well combined.

Spread the granola in the baking pans and bake for 50–60 minutes, until dry and lightly browned. Remove from the oven and let cool. When cool, crumble the granola into large pieces with your hands. Mix in the optional currants or raisins. Stored in airtight containers, mason jars, or ziplock bags in the freezer, the granola will keep for 6 months. It will remain fresh and crispy and doesn't need to be thawed before using.

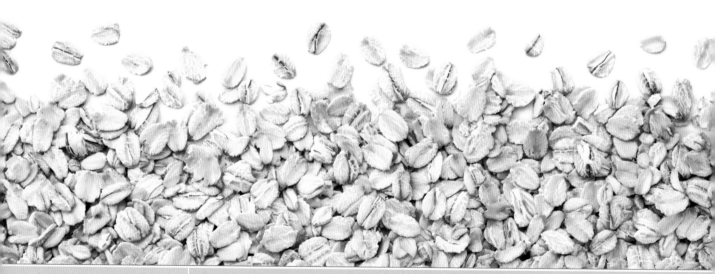

GOLDEN Scrambled Tofu and Veggies

Top this protein feast with hot sauce, salsa, or diced avocado. Turmeric, the main spice in curry powder, is well known for its anti-inflammatory properties. It adds a beautiful yellow hue to food, and in this dish it works perfectly to mimic the color of scrambled eggs.

1 package (12 oz./360 g) firm or medium-firm tofu, drained and patted dry

1 tablespoon (15 ml) low-sodium or regular tamari

¼ teaspoon (1 ml) ground turmeric

2 tablespoons (30 ml) low-sodium or regular vegetable broth or water

1 cup (250 ml) sliced mushrooms

½ cup (125 ml) sliced red bell pepper

¼ cup (60 ml) sliced green onions

2 cloves garlic, minced

2 cups (500 ml) chopped dark leafy greens (such as spinach, bok choy, or kale), packed

2 tablespoons (30 ml) chopped fresh herbs (such as parsley, basil, or oregano), or 2 teaspoons (10 ml) dried herbs

2 tablespoons (30 ml) nutritional yeast flakes

Freshly ground black pepper

Crumble the tofu into a medium bowl. Alternatively, for a finer texture, mash the tofu with a fork or potato masher in a medium bowl. Add the tamari and turmeric and stir until evenly distributed. Set aside.

Put the broth in a large skillet over medium-high heat. Add the mushrooms, bell pepper, green onions, and garlic. Cook, stirring frequently, until the vegetables are tender, about 5 minutes. Add a little more broth, if needed, to prevent sticking.

Add the tofu to the vegetables and cook, stirring frequently, until the consistency resembles scrambled eggs, about 5 minutes.

Add the greens and herbs and cook, stirring constantly, until the greens are wilted, about 2 minutes. Remove from the heat, stir in the nutritional yeast, and season with pepper to taste. Serve warm.

SERVING SUGGESTION: To round out the meal, serve the scramble with cooked sweet potatoes or whole-grain toast on the side. Alternatively, fill whole-grain tortillas or wraps with the scramble to make satisfying breakfast burritos.

Per one-half recipe (313 ml):

Calories: 206

Protein: 23 g

Leucine: 1,600 mg

Fat: 10 g

Carbohydrate: 11 g

Fiber: 9 g

Minerals:

Iron: 5.8 mg

Zinc: 2.9 mg

Calcium: 553 mg*

Sodium: 595 mg

Percent of calories from:

Protein 41%

Fat 39%

Carbohydrate 20%

*Check tofu labels for calcium content. Some brands and types are very rich in calcium.

TEMPTING Tempeh

Tempeh is a versatile soy food that originates from Indonesia. Its texture has been described as meaty and its taste as nutty. Cooking it in broth or water or steaming it allows the marinade to penetrate it better. Tempeh works well in stir-fries, The Big Bowl (page 164), Gado Gado (page 169), and sandwiches. It also can be crumbled into dishes to resemble ground meat.

8 ounces (240 g) tempeh

2 cups (500 ml) low-sodium or regular vegetable broth or water

2 teaspoons (10 ml) low-sodium or regular tamari

Seasoning blend of your choice

Cut the tempeh into slices, strips, or cubes ½ inch (1.5 cm) thick. Put the broth in a medium-size saucepan and bring to a boil over medium-high heat. Add the tempeh, decrease the heat to medium-low, and simmer for 10 minutes. Remove the tempeh from the broth using a slotted spoon and arrange the tempeh on a medium plate or tray.

Sprinkle, spray, or brush each strip with the tamari on both sides and sprinkle on the seasoning mix of your choice.

Heat a medium-size nonstick grill pan or skillet over medium heat. Place the tempeh on the grill and cook until the first side starts to brown, 2 to 3 minutes. Flip the tempeh over and cook the other side until lightly browned, about 2 minutes.

TIP: Save the simmer broth for soup or to cook rice.

MISO-MUSTARD TEMPEH: Put 2 tablespoons (30 ml) miso (any color), 2 tablespoons (30 ml) Dijon or grainy mustard, 2 tablespoons (30 ml) low-sodium or regular tamari, and 2 teaspoons (10 ml) toasted sesame oil (optional) in a medium flat-bottomed bowl and whisk until well combined. After removing the tempeh from the broth, dip it into this marinade and turn to coat both sides. Let the tempeh marinate for 10 minutes, then cook as directed.

TEMPEH SANDWICH: Spread your favorite bread, fresh or toasted, with mustard or vegan mayonnaise and add the tempeh. Top the tempeh with one or more of the following options: vegan cheese, avocado, tomato slices, lettuce, arugula, baby spinach, or drained sauerkraut. Serve as is or grill in a medium skillet over medium-high heat or in a panini pan until browned, about 3 minutes per side. If desired, brush the outside of the bread with a little olive oil or vegan butter before grilling.

Per one-half recipe, or ¾ cup (185 ml):

Calories: 193

Protein: 22 g

Leucine 1,679 mg

Fat: 6 g

Carbohydrate: 14 g

Fiber: 10 g

Minerals:

Iron: 2.6 mg

Zinc: 1.3 mg

Calcium: 82 mg

Sodium: 354 mg

Percent of calories from:

Protein 45%

Fat 27%

Carbohydrate 28%

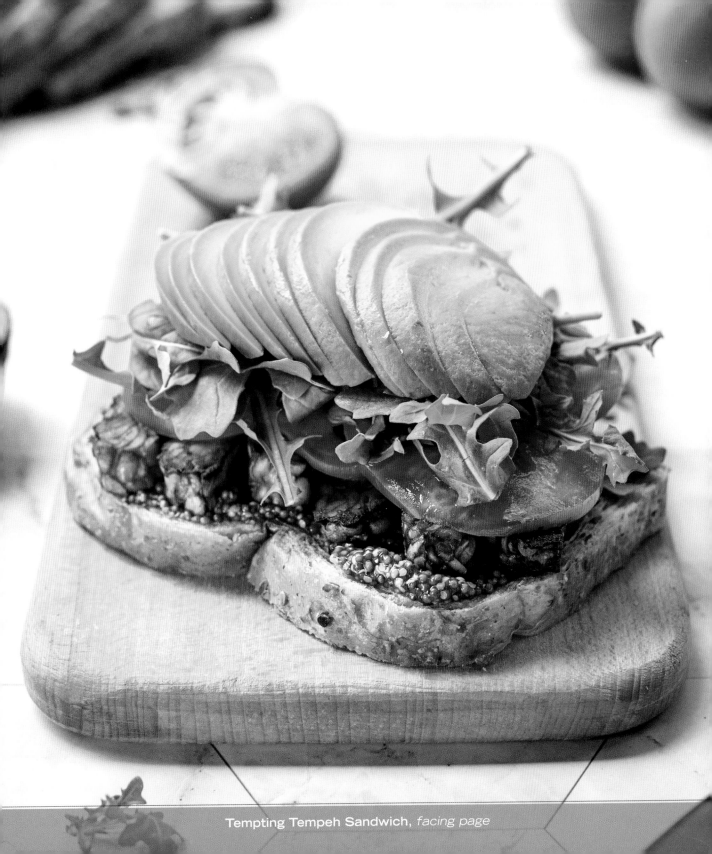

Tempting Tempeh Sandwich, *facing page*

TASTY Tofu Fingers

These tofu fingers can be sprinkled on a salad or stir-fry, enjoyed as a snack, or prepared as slices and used in a sandwich. They can be breaded or unbreaded and cooked in myriad ways, depending on your preferences.

1 package (12 oz./360 g) extra-firm or firm tofu

⅓ cup (85 ml) low-sodium or regular tamari or soy sauce

2 tablespoons (30 ml) minced or grated fresh ginger

2 tablespoons (30 ml) toasted sesame oil

1 tablespoon (15 ml) unseasoned rice vinegar or apple cider vinegar

2 cloves garlic, minced

Cut the tofu into fingers that are 2 x ½ x ½ inches (5 x 1.5 x 1.5 cm). Set aside.

Put marinade ingredients in a bowl with a lid. Add the tofu fingers and marinate for at least 15 minutes at room temperature or 8–12 hours in the refrigerator (the longer marinating time will allow the tofu to absorb more flavor from the marinade). Gently stir a couple of times so all of the tofu pieces come into contact with the marinade. Lift the tofu pieces from the marinade using a slotted spoon (store the leftover marinade in a sealed container in the refrigerator to use another time). Cook the tofu fingers using one of the following methods for the time suggested or until lightly browned.

COOKING METHODS: Put the marinated, drained, and optionally coated tofu pieces in one of the following.

- **An air fryer.** Air-fry at 375 degrees F (190 degrees C) for 15 minutes.
- **An oven preheated to 350 degrees F (177 degrees C).** Line a medium baking sheet with a silicone baking mat or parchment paper. Alternatively, oil the baking sheet. Arrange the tofu on the prepared baking sheet and bake for 20 minutes, or until the tofu is lightly browned and crispy.
- **A large skillet over medium heat.** Coat the skillet with a thin layer of oil, decrease the heat to low, and cook the tofu, turning it frequently, until lightly browned on each side, about 5 minutes.

Per one-third recipe, or ⅔ cup (170 ml)*:
Calories: 206
Protein: 21 g
Leucine: 1,644 mg
Fat: 13 g
Carbohydrate: 4 g
Fiber: 3 g

Minerals:
Iron: 3.5 mg
Zinc: 1.8 mg
Calcium: 798 mg**
Sodium: 463 mg

Percent of calories from:
Protein 39%
Fat 53%
Carbohydrate 8%

*Based on the unbreaded version and using one-third of the marinade for the analysis.

**Check tofu labels for calcium content. Some brands and types are very rich in calcium.

COATED TOFU FINGERS: Put ¼ cup (60 ml) of nutritional yeast flakes or fine bread crumbs in a medium bowl. Add dried herbs, spices, or your favorite seasoning blend for a flavor boost. Gently coat all sides of the tofu fingers. Add a little more breading if needed. Cook the tofu fingers by one of the methods above for the time listed or until lightly browned.

SUPER-SPEEDY TOFU FINGERS: Dip extra-firm tofu slices or fingers briefly in tamari, soy sauce, or Bragg Liquid Aminos and then into nutritional yeast flakes. If you like, add a sprinkle of your favorite seasoning to the yeast. Then, sauté the tofu in a little oil or cook it using one of the other methods above.

NUTRITION NOTES: The protein per serving can vary (from slightly to significantly), depending on the type of tofu used.

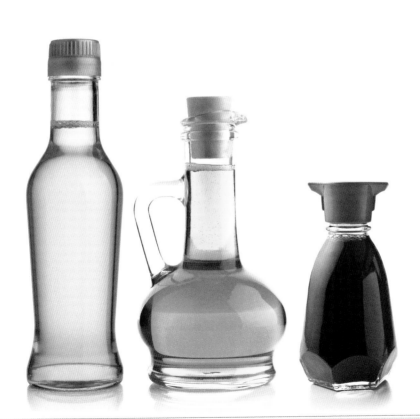

CREAMY Vanilla Chia Pudding

Chia pudding can serve as an everyday dessert or a creamy addition to a breakfast bowl. This version gets a substantial protein boost with hemp seeds and protein-rich nondairy milk. Blending the hemp seeds with the milk makes the pudding extra creamy.

3 cups (750 ml) fortified unsweetened protein-rich nondairy milk (such as soy or pea)

½ cup (125 ml) hemp seeds

4 pitted medjool dates, or 12 pitted deglet noor dates

1 teaspoon (5 ml) vanilla extract

⅓ cup (85 ml) chia seeds

Put the milk, hemp seeds, dates, and vanilla extract in a blender and process on high speed until smooth.

Add the chia seeds and pulse once or twice, just to distribute the chia seeds through the liquid. Pour into a medium bowl or glass jar, cover, and refrigerate for 30–60 minutes.

After the pudding has chilled, stir it with a spoon, table knife, or whisk to remove any lumps and distribute the chia seeds evenly. Refrigerate for at least 4 hours before serving. Stored in an airtight container in the refrigerator, the pudding will keep for 5 days.

NUTRITION NOTES: Using fortified milk will add vitamin D and calcium. The hemp and chia seeds provide 5.1 grams of omega-3 fatty acids.

SERVING SUGGESTION: Serve with fresh fruit, berries, stewed fruit, unsweetened shredded dried coconut, chopped raw nuts, raw seeds, or other toppings of your choice.

CHOCOLATE CHIA PUDDING: Add 3 tablespoons (45 ml) unsweetened cocoa powder. Increase the dates to 6 pitted medjool or 18 pitted deglet noor dates. Add the cocoa powder at the same time as the milk, hemp seeds, dates, and vanilla extract. For a flavor boost, add a pinch of salt and a sprinkle of ground cinnamon. Proceed with the basic recipe.

MASON JAR PARFAITS: Alternate layers of chia pudding with fruit (berries, chopped fresh fruit, stewed fruit, or a combination) and your choice of chopped raw nuts, raw seeds, unsweetened shredded dried coconut, granola, or a combination.

Per 1 cup (250 ml):
Calories: 474
Protein: 17 g
Leucine: 1,010 mg
Fat: 18 g
Carbohydrate: 69 g
Fiber: 12 g

Minerals:
Iron: 4.6 mg
Zinc: 3 mg
Calcium: 196 mg
Sodium: 108 mg

Percent of calories from:
Protein 14%
Fat 32%
Carbohydrate 54%

Double-Chocolate Surprise COOKIES

These tasty treats are higher in protein than most cookies, and they even provide iron and zinc. The surprise ingredient is black beans!

1½ cups (375 ml) cooked or canned black beans, drained and rinsed

1 cup (250 ml) pitted soft dates, packed (see tip)

½ cup (125 ml) unsweetened peanut butter, nut butter, or seed butter

¼ cup (60 ml) unsweetened cocoa powder

3 tablespoons (45 ml) hemp seeds

2 tablespoons (30 ml) ground flaxseeds

1 teaspoon (5 ml) vanilla extract

½ teaspoon (2 ml) salt

½ cup (125 ml) coarsely chopped walnuts

½ cup (125 ml) dark chocolate chunks or chips

Preheat the oven to 350 degrees F (177 degrees C). Line 2 medium baking sheets with silicone baking mats or parchment paper. Alternatively, mist the baking sheets with cooking spray.

Put the beans, dates, peanut butter, cocoa powder, hemp seeds, flaxseeds, vanilla extract, and salt in a food processor and process until smooth. Add the walnuts and chocolate chunks and pulse just until evenly distributed. Form the dough into balls using 1 heaping tablespoon of dough per ball. Put 12 balls on each prepared baking sheet. Flatten the balls slightly so the cookies are about ½ inch (1.5 cm) thick. Bake for 12–14 minutes, or until very lightly browned on the bottoms. Let the cookies cool before serving or storing. Stored in an airtight container, the cookies will keep for 3 days at room temperature and 4 months in the freezer.

TIP: If the dates you have are hard, steam them briefly until they soften.

VARIATIONS: To add a little pizzazz, top each cookie with a pecan half before baking, or drizzle the baked cookies with 1–2 ounces (30–60 g) of melted chocolate after they have cooled. The dates may be replaced with ½ cup (125 ml) natural maple syrup.

Per 2 cookies:
Calories: 229
Protein: 7 g
Leucine: 500 mg
Fat: 14 g
Carbohydrate: 25 g
Fiber: 5 g

Minerals:
Iron: 1.7 mg
Zinc: 1.3 mg
Calcium: 31 mg
Sodium: 129 mg

Percent of calories from:
Protein 12%
Fat 49%
Carbohydrate 39%

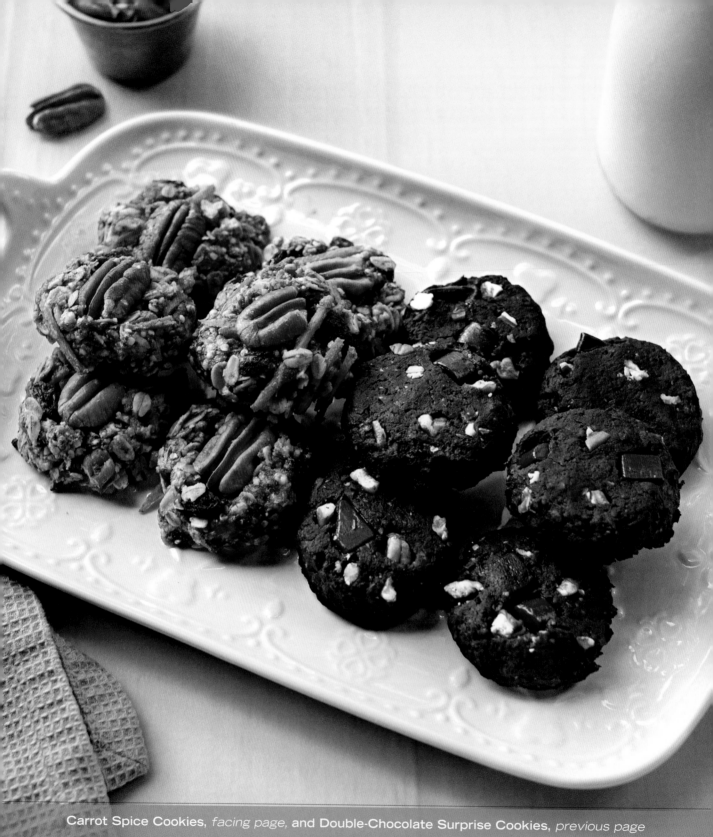

Carrot Spice Cookies, *facing page*, and Double-Chocolate Surprise Cookies, *previous page*

Carrot Spice COOKIES

These cookies are nutritious enough to eat for breakfast and also make a great anytime pick-me-up.

1 cup (250 ml) pitted dates, packed

⅓ cup (85 ml) water

¾ cup (185 ml) cashew butter, almond butter, or mixed nut-and-seed butter (see tip)

¼ cup (60 ml) hemp seeds

2 tablespoons (30 ml) ground flaxseeds

1 tablespoon (15 ml) pumpkin pie spice (see sidebar)

1 teaspoon (5 ml) vanilla extract

½ teaspoon (2 ml) salt

1 cup (250 ml) grated carrots, packed

1 cup (250 ml) old-fashioned rolled oats

1 cup (250 ml) walnuts or pecans or a mix of both, coarsely chopped

½ cup (125 ml) raisins

36 pecan halves (optional)

Preheat the oven to 325 degrees F (163 degrees C). Line 3 large baking sheets with silicone baking mats or parchment paper. Alternatively, lightly spray the baking sheets with vegetable oil.

Put the dates and water in a small saucepan. Cover and cook over low heat until the dates are soft, about 5 minutes. Mash the dates with a potato masher.

Put the mashed dates, cashew butter, hemp seeds, flaxseeds, pumpkin pie spice, vanilla extract, and salt in a large bowl. Stir until well combined. Stir in the carrots and oats, then fold in the walnuts and raisins.

Drop the dough by heaping tablespoons on the baking sheets, putting 12 cookies on each baking sheet. Use a second spoon to help get the dough off the first spoon. Shape the cookies with your hands to form nice round cookie shapes if needed. Press an optional pecan half on top of each cookie. Bake for 25–30 minutes, or until the cookies are lightly browned on the bottom.

Remove the cookies from the oven, let cool, and store in an airtight container. To help maintain freshness, leave out only what you will use within 1–2 days. Freeze the rest.

NUTRITION NOTES: Seeds and cashews provide zinc as well as iron.

TIP: If your nut butter is quite firm, add 1 tablespoon (15 ml) of a neutral-tasting vegetable oil (such as avocado oil) to thin it.

HOMEMADE PUMPKIN PIE SPICE

Makes 1 tablespoon (15 ml)

1½ teaspoons (7 ml) ground cinnamon

½ teaspoon (2 ml) ground ginger

½ teaspoon (2 ml) ground nutmeg

¼ teaspoon (1 ml) ground cloves

¼ teaspoon (1 ml) ground allspice

Put all the ingredients in a small jar, seal tightly, and shake well to thoroughly combine.

Per 3 cookies:
Calories: 275
Protein: 7 g
Leucine: 590 mg
Fat: 17 g
Carbohydrate: 28 g
Fiber: 4 g

Minerals:
Iron: 2 mg
Zinc: 1.6 mg
Calcium: 38 mg
Sodium: 90 mg

Percent of calories from:
Protein 10%
Fat 53%
Carbohydrate 37%

Power Greens SALAD

This recipe will train your brain to view salad as a satisfying main dish. When you are ready to eat, top the greens with two protein boosts plus your choice of optional additions for color and protective antioxidants and phytochemicals.

GREENS

4 cups (1 L) romaine lettuce or mixed greens, torn into bite-size pieces

2 cups (500 ml) stemmed and thinly sliced kale, packed

2 cups (500 ml) thinly sliced napa cabbage or collard greens

PROTEIN BOOSTS

4 ounces (120 g) Tasty Tofu Fingers (pages 132–133) or Tempting Tempeh (page 130)

4 ounces (120 g) baked or smoked tofu or tempeh, cubed

1 cup (250 ml) cooked or canned chickpeas, other beans, or lentils, drained and rinsed

1 cup (250 ml) edamame or green chickpeas, prepared as directed on package

7 falafel patties (120 g total) or other veggie balls

4 ounces (120 g) vegan chicken or beef

OPTIONAL ADDITIONS

Sliced avocado, tomato, radishes, or red onion

Grated carrots or beets

Chopped cucumber, bell peppers, or zucchini

Broccoli or cauliflower florets

Sprouts or microgreens

Sugar snap peas

Corn kernels

Sautéed mushrooms

Cooked quinoa, wild rice, Kamut, or other whole grain

Cooked and cubed sweet potato, yam, white potato, or squash

Seeds or nuts

Vegan feta or other vegan cheese, crumbled or cubed

Lemon-Tahini Protein-Plus Dressing (page 148) or dressing of choice

Per one-half recipe*:
Calories: 225
Protein: 16 g
Leucine: 1,110 mg
Fat: 6 g
Carbohydrate: 30 g
Fiber: 10 g

Minerals:
Iron: 4.8 mg
Zinc: 2.2 mg
Calcium: 310 mg**
Sodium: 33 mg

Percent of calories from:
Protein 27%
Fat 22%
Carbohydrate 51%

*Based on 4 cups (1 L) greens plus 4 ounces (120 g) firm tofu and 1 cup (250 ml) chickpeas. Analysis does not include the dressing, which will deliver additional protein.

**Check tofu labels. Calcium content varies widely depending on tofu brand and type.

Put the lettuce, kale, and cabbage in a large bowl and toss to mix. Just before serving, add 2 or more protein boosts and top with your choice of optional additions. Add the dressing and toss until evenly distributed.

TIP: For an instant salad, double or triple the amount of greens and store in a large, tightly sealed container in the refrigerator. The greens will keep for 4 days.

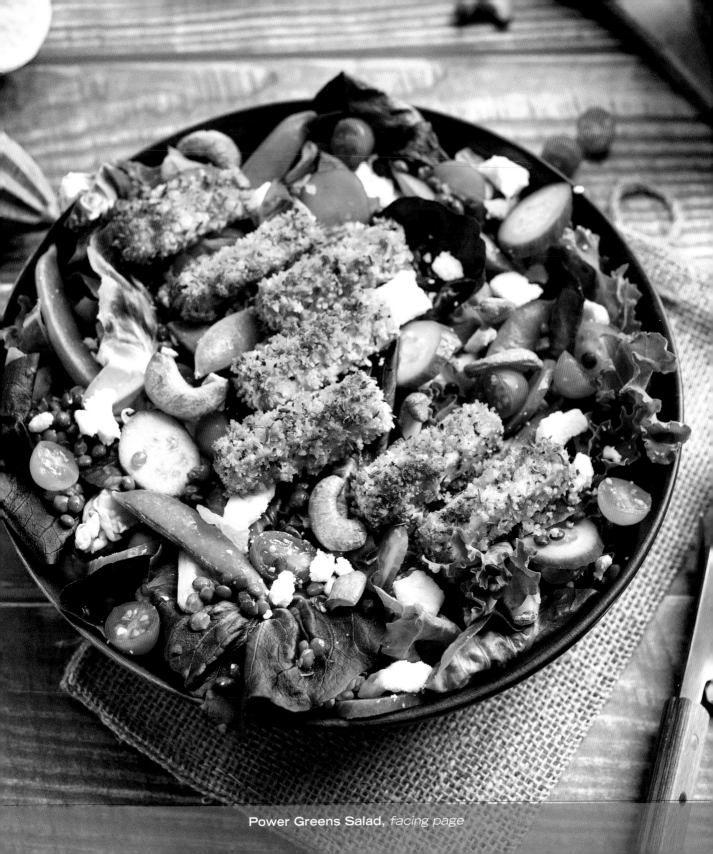

Power Greens Salad, *facing page*

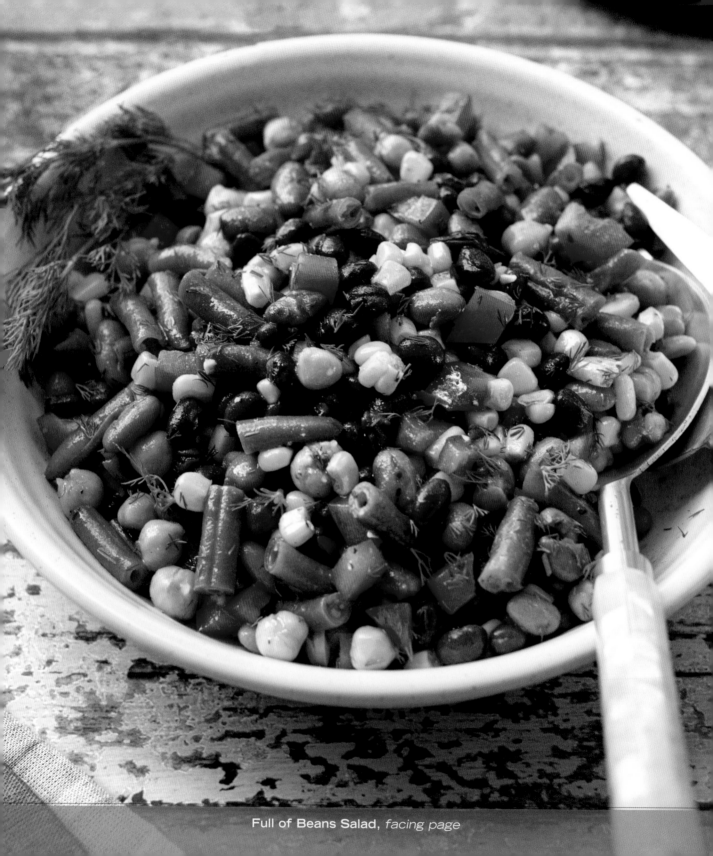

Full of Beans Salad, *facing page*

Full of Beans SALAD

For this colorful salad, experiment with a variety of cooked or canned beans—such as black beans, cannellini beans, chickpeas, edamame, lima beans, navy beans, pinto beans, and red beans—and include two or more types. Feel free to increase the amount or variety of vegetables in this salad. Swap the red bell pepper and corn for other vegetables, such as steamed asparagus, broccoli, cauliflower, or green beans or fresh cherry tomatoes, thinly sliced greens, or snow peas.

MARINADE

¼ cup (60 ml) freshly squeezed lime or lemon juice or vinegar of choice

2 tablespoons (30 ml) olive oil or sesame oil (optional)

2 teaspoons (10 ml) natural maple syrup (optional)

3 tablespoons (45 ml) chopped fresh dill or cilantro, or 1 tablespoon (15 ml) dried dill weed or cilantro

1 teaspoon (5 ml) Dijon mustard

1 teaspoon (5 ml) minced garlic, or ¼ teaspoon (1 ml) garlic powder

¼ teaspoon (1 ml) salt, plus more as needed

¼ teaspoon (1 ml) freshly ground black pepper, plus more as needed

SALAD

3 cups (750 ml) cooked or canned beans, drained and rinsed

1 cup (250 ml) chopped red bell pepper

1 cup (250 ml) frozen corn, thawed, or canned corn, drained

To make the marinade, put the lime juice, optional oil, optional maple syrup, dill, mustard, garlic, salt, and pepper in a small jar. Seal tightly and shake until well combined.

To make the salad, put the beans, red bell pepper, and corn in a large bowl. Add the marinade and gently toss. Marinate for at least 3 hours in the refrigerator, stirring occasionally. Taste and add more salt or pepper as needed. Stored in a sealed container in the refrigerator, the salad will keep for 4 days.

Per 1 cup (250 ml)*:
Calories: 192
Protein: 11 g
Leucine: 900 mg
Fat: 1 g
Carbohydrate: 37 g
Fiber: 11 g

Minerals:
Iron: 2.8 mg
Zinc: 1.5 mg
Calcium: 46 mg
Sodium: 123 mg

Percent of calories from:
Protein 22%
Fat 4%
Carbohydrate 74%

*Based on black beans, pinto beans, baby lima beans, red bell pepper, and corn.

LENTIL Tabbouleh

This recipe is inspired by a dish that has served as a dietary staple in Lebanon since the Middle Ages. In its traditional form, tabbouleh is made with bulgur. In this protein-packed variation, the bulgur is replaced by lentils.

4 cups (1 L) water

1 cup (250 ml) small lentils (such as black beluga, French, or small brown)

2 cups (500 ml) minced fresh parsley, packed

2 firm tomatoes, chopped, or 2 cups (475 ml) halved or quartered cherry tomatoes

1½ cups (375 ml) chopped cucumber

½ cup (125 ml) chopped fresh mint leaves

⅓ cup (85 ml) freshly squeezed lemon juice

2 tablespoons (30 ml) olive oil

3 cloves garlic, minced

¾ teaspoon (4 ml) salt

Bring the water to a boil in a medium saucepan over high heat. Add the lentils, then decrease the heat to low. Cook until the lentils are soft, about 30 minutes. Drain the lentils and rinse them with cold water.

Put the cooled lentils, parsley, tomatoes, cucumber, and mint in a large bowl. Put the lemon juice, olive oil, garlic, and salt in a small bowl and stir vigorously. Pour the dressing over the salad ingredients and toss gently. Stored in a sealed container in the refrigerator, the salad will keep for 2 days.

Per 1½ cups (375 ml):
Calories: 238
Protein: 13 g
Leucine: 870 mg
Fat: 7 g
Carbohydrate: 35 g
Fiber: 7 g

Minerals:
Iron: 5 mg
Zinc: 1.9 mg
Calcium: 82 mg
Sodium: 433 mg

Percent of calories from:
Protein 20%
Fat 24%
Carbohydrate 56%

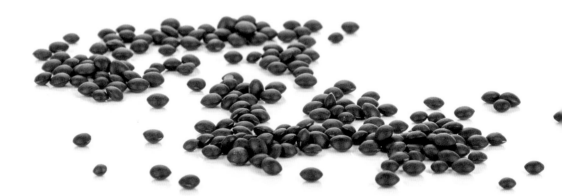

Kale Salad WITH ORANGE-GINGER DRESSING

If you have been at a loss as to what to do with kale, here is a simple solution. Ginger lovers, this dressing is amazing!

SALAD

6 cups (1.5 L) stemmed and thinly sliced kale

1 cup (250 ml) thinly sliced red cabbage

1 carrot, grated or julienned

½ red bell pepper, thinly sliced

2 tablespoons (30 ml) chopped fresh mint, or 2 teaspoons (10 ml) dried mint

¼ cup (60 ml) raw pumpkin seeds, sunflower seeds, or hemp seeds

ORANGE-GINGER DRESSING

⅔ cup (170 ml) freshly squeezed orange juice

¼ cup (60 ml) tahini

2 pitted medjool dates, or 6 pitted deglet noor dates

2 tablespoons (30 ml) low-sodium or regular tamari, Bragg Liquid Aminos, soy sauce, or miso (any color)

2 tablespoons (30 ml) chopped fresh ginger

1 tablespoon (15 ml) apple cider vinegar or freshly squeezed lemon juice

Cayenne or freshly ground black pepper

To make the salad, put the kale, cabbage, carrot, red bell pepper, and mint in a large bowl, and toss to mix.

To make the orange-ginger dressing, put the orange juice, tahini, dates, tamari, ginger, and vinegar in a blender. Process until smooth. Season with cayenne to taste. Pour the dressing over the salad, and toss until evenly distributed. Let marinate at room temperature or in the refrigerator for at least 20 minutes before serving. Sprinkle with the pumpkin seeds just before serving. Stored in a sealed container in the refrigerator, the salad (without the seeds) will keep for 3 days (add the seeds just before serving).

Per 2 cups (500 ml):
Calories: 306
Protein: 11 g
Leucine: 717 mg
Fat: 17 g
Carbohydrate: 33 g
Fiber: 6 g

Minerals:
Iron: 3.4 mg
Zinc: 2.3 mg
Calcium: 124 mg
Sodium: 517 mg

Percent of calories from:
Protein 14%
Fat 46%
Carbohydrate 40%

PEANUT-EDAMAME Noodle Salad

Pasta salads are perfect for picnics and potlucks as they hold up well. The napa cabbage can be replaced with Asian greens, thinly sliced kale, or spinach, and the green onions with sweet or red onions. Vary the colors of peppers, and add other veggies such as grated daikon, shredded red cabbage, or cucumber strips. Replace edamame with baked or smoked tofu. If you like spicy foods, increase the hot sauce.

PEANUT DRESSING

⅓ cup (85 ml) water

½ cup (125 ml) peanut butter

¼ cup (60 ml) freshly squeezed lime juice

2 tablespoons (30 ml) unseasoned rice vinegar

1½ tablespoons (22 ml) low-sodium or regular tamari or Bragg Liquid Aminos

1 tablespoon (15 ml) grated fresh ginger

2 cloves garlic, minced

1 teaspoon (5 ml) toasted sesame oil

1 teaspoon (5 ml) chili sauce, hot sauce, or sriracha sauce, or pinch cayenne

SALAD

5 ounces (150 g) dry edamame noodles, soba (buckwheat) noodles, or other noodles

1½ cups (375 ml) frozen shelled edamame, peas, or green chickpeas

2 cups (500 ml) thinly sliced napa cabbage (or other greens), packed

2 carrots, shredded or grated

1 red bell pepper, thinly sliced

½ cup (125 ml) chopped fresh cilantro, parsley, or basil (or a combination)

2 green onions, thinly sliced

¼ cup (60 ml) roasted unsalted peanuts, whole or coarsely chopped

Per 2 cups (500 ml):
Calories: 495
Protein: 34 g
Leucine: 2,299 mg
Fat: 29 g
Carbohydrate: 36 g
Fiber: 16 g

Minerals:
Iron: 7.4 mg
Zinc: 3.1 mg
Calcium: 215 mg
Sodium: 592 mg

Percent of calories from:
Protein 25%
Fat 48%
Carbohydrate 27%

To make the peanut dressing, put the water, peanut butter, lime juice, vinegar, tamari, ginger, garlic, sesame oil, and chili sauce in a medium bowl or jar and whisk until smooth.

To make the salad, prepare the noodles and edamame according to package directions. Strain the noodles and rinse with cold water. Drain the edamame and rinse with cold water.

Put the noodles and edamame in a large bowl. Add the napa cabbage, carrots, red bell pepper, cilantro, and green onions. Pour the dressing on top and gently toss to combine the ingredients. Sprinkle the peanuts on top just before serving.

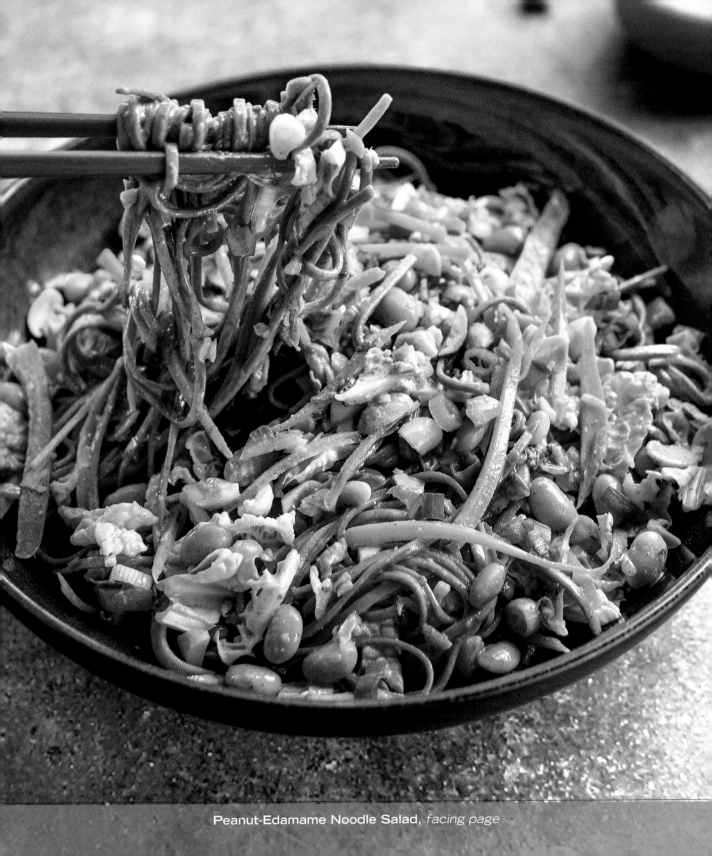

Peanut-Edamame Noodle Salad, *facing page*

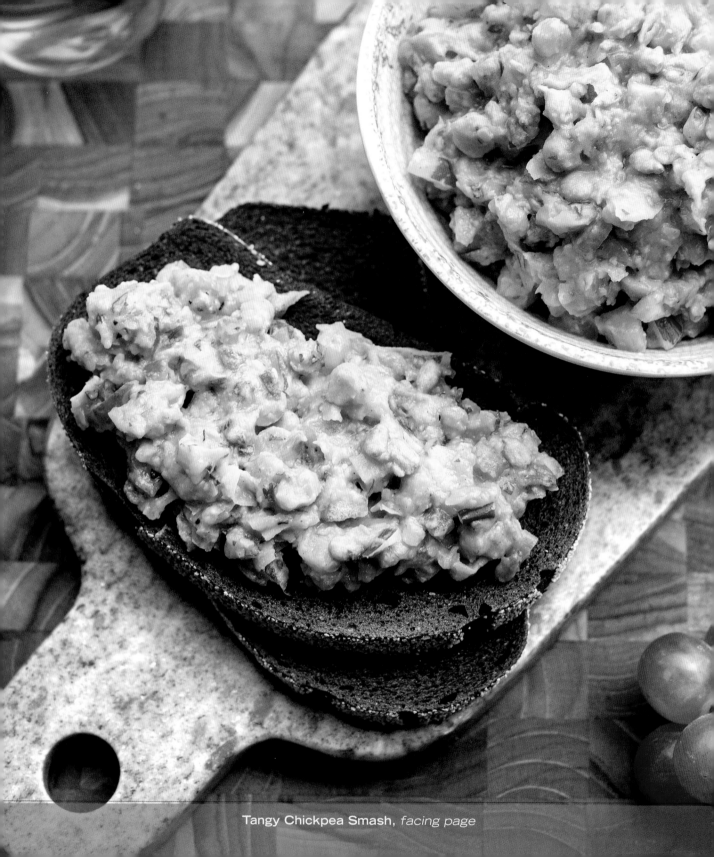

Tangy Chickpea Smash, *facing page*

Tangy Chickpea SMASH

This sandwich or wrap filling is reminiscent of tuna salad, especially with the addition of kelp or dulse. This also is a good addition to a green salad. The optional additions provide extra flavor and a nutrition boost. The seaweed adds iodine, the nutritional yeast flakes supply vitamin B_{12}, and the sunflower seeds provide vitamin E.

CHICKPEA SMASH

1 can (14–16 oz./398–454 ml) chickpeas, drained and rinsed

¼ cup (60 ml) minced sweet or red onion

1 stalk celery, diced

1 large dill pickle, diced

2 tablespoons (30 ml) chopped fresh dill or parsley, or 2 teaspoons (10 ml) dried

OPTIONAL ADDITIONS

2 tablespoons (30 ml) unsalted roasted or raw sunflower seeds

1 tablespoon (15 ml) nutritional yeast flakes

¼ teaspoon (1 ml) kelp powder, or 1 teaspoon (5 ml) dulse flakes

DRESSING

3 tablespoons (45 ml) tahini

3 tablespoons (45 ml) freshly squeezed lemon juice

1 teaspoon (5 ml) Dijon mustard

¼ teaspoon (1 ml) salt

Freshly ground black pepper

Per ½ cup (125 ml):
Calories: 188
Protein: 8 g
Leucine: 576 mg
Fat: 8 g
Carbohydrate: 23 g
Fiber: 6 g

Minerals:
Iron: 2.5 mg
Zinc: 1.6 mg
Calcium: 75 mg
Sodium: 439 mg

Percent of calories from:
Protein 17%
Fat 36%
Carbohydrate 47%

To make the chickpea smash, put the chickpeas in a medium bowl and mash them (a potato masher works well for this).

Stir in the onion, celery, pickle, and dill plus any optional additions.

To make the dressing, combine the tahini, lemon juice, mustard, and salt in a small bowl. Stir the dressing into the chickpea filling until thoroughly combined. Season with pepper to taste. Stored in a sealed container in the refrigerator, the salad will keep for 3 days.

TIP: If you do not have lemons or their juice handy, substitute lime juice or apple cider vinegar.

Lemon-Tahini PROTEIN-PLUS DRESSING

Unlike most oil- or sugar-based salad dressings, this one is made of whole foods! It adds protein to salads, steamed broccoli or cauliflower, and baked potatoes. For the best flavor, use freshly squeezed juice. Nutritional yeast makes this an excellent source of B vitamins, including B_{12}, and hemp seeds provide omega-3 fatty acids and zinc.

1 cup (250 ml) water

⅓ cup (85 ml) nutritional yeast flakes

⅓ cup (85 ml) hemp seeds

⅓ cup (85 ml) tahini

⅓ cup (85 ml) freshly squeezed lemon or lime juice or apple cider vinegar

1 tablespoon (15 ml) Dijon or stone-ground mustard

2 cloves garlic

½ teaspoon (2 ml) salt

Put the water, nutritional yeast flakes, hemp seeds, tahini, lemon juice, mustard, garlic, and salt in a blender and process for 30 seconds, or until smooth. Taste the dressing and add more salt if needed. Stored in a sealed container in the refrigerator, the dressing will keep for 2 weeks.

SWEET LEMON-TAHINI DRESSING: If you prefer a sweeter dressing, blend in 2 or 3 pitted dates or 1 tablespoon (15 ml) of natural maple syrup.

Per ⅓ cup (85 ml):
Calories: 167
Protein: 9 g
Leucine: 591 mg
Fat: 13 g
Carbohydrate: 8 g
Fiber: 1 g

Minerals:
Iron: 1.7 mg
Zinc: 2.8 mg
Calcium: 35 mg
Sodium: 227 mg

Percent of calories from:
Protein 19%
Fat 63%
Carbohydrate 18%

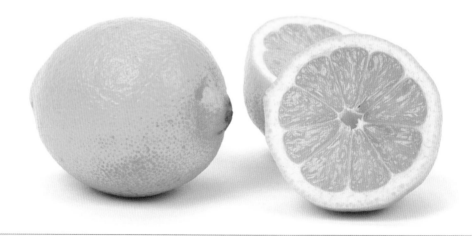

Hummus and Lime DRESSING

For a quick, easy, and protein-rich dressing, all you need is a container of hummus and a lime or two. If you prefer, replace lime with lemon or a favorite vinegar. Add herbs or spices to suit your palate.

¼ cup (60 ml) water, plus more as needed

½ cup (125 ml) hummus, any flavor

2 tablespoons (30 ml) freshly squeezed lime juice

½ teaspoon (2 ml) ground turmeric

Put the water in a blender. Add the hummus, lime juice, and turmeric. Blend until smooth. Alternatively, you can mix these ingredients in a small bowl with a whisk or fork.

TIP: For a slightly thinner dressing, add additional water, 1 tablespoon (15 ml) at a time, until the desired consistency is achieved.

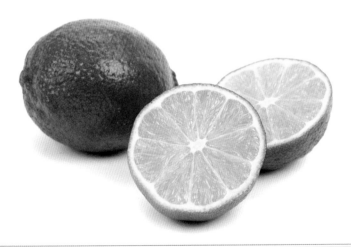

Per ⅓ cup (85 ml):
Calories: 90
Protein: 4 g
Leucine: 183 mg
Fat: 5 g
Carbohydrate: 9 g
Fiber: 3 g

Minerals:
Iron: 1.7 mg
Zinc: 1 mg
Calcium: 24 mg
Sodium: 194 mg

Percent of calories from:
Protein 17%
Fat 46%
Carbohydrate 37%

Ginger, Lime, and Miso DRESSING

MAKES 1 ⅓ CUPS (335 ML)

This dressing is perfect for dinner bowls or salads.

⅓ cup (85 ml) fortified unsweetened coconut milk, other fortified unsweetened nondairy milk, or canned coconut milk

¼ cup (60 ml) cashew, almond, or sunflower seed butter

3 tablespoons (45 ml) unseasoned rice vinegar

3 tablespoons (45 ml) freshly squeezed lime juice

2 tablespoons (30 ml) miso (any color)

1½ tablespoons (22 ml) low-sodium or regular tamari

1 pitted medjool date, or 3 pitted deglet noor dates

1 tablespoon (15 ml) chopped fresh ginger

2 cloves garlic

Put the milk, cashew butter, vinegar, lime juice, miso, tamari, date, ginger, and garlic in a blender and process on high speed until smooth and creamy. Stored in a tightly sealed container in the refrigerator, the dressing will keep for 1 week.

TIP: If the dressing is too thick (which may happen after it's been stored in the refrigerator), thin it with 1 tablespoon (15 ml) of nondairy milk or more as needed.

VARIATION: Replace the dates with 2 teaspoons (10 ml) natural maple syrup.

Per ⅓ cup (85 ml):
Calories: 146
Protein: 5 g
Leucine: 326 mg
Fat: 9 g
Carbohydrate: 13 g
Fiber: 1 g

Minerals:
Iron: 1.4 mg
Zinc: 1.1 mg
Calcium: 47 mg
Sodium: 602 mg

Percent of calories from:
Protein 13%
Fat 52%
Carbohydrate 35%

Gado Gado SAUCE

This spicy peanut sauce is the topping for Gado Gado (page 169). However, it also pairs perfectly with salads, power bowls, and wraps. Tahini replaces the more traditional sesame oil used in peanut sauce, and dates replace the sugar.

¾ cup (185 ml) very hot water

½ cup (125 ml) peanut butter

2 pitted medjool dates, or 6 pitted deglet noor dates

2 tablespoons (30 ml) freshly squeezed lime juice

2 tablespoons (30 ml) tahini

1 tablespoon (15 ml) low-sodium or regular tamari

1 teaspoon (5 ml) tamarind paste (optional)

1 tablespoon (15 ml) chopped fresh ginger

2 cloves garlic

2 small hot chiles, or ½ teaspoon (2 ml) hot sauce

Put the water, peanut butter, dates, lime juice, tahini, tamari, optional tamarind paste, ginger, garlic, and hot chiles in a blender and process on high speed until smooth. Use immediately or chill before serving. Stored in a sealed container in the refrigerator, the sauce will keep for 5 days.

TIP: Although the tamarind paste is optional, it gives this sauce a more authentic flavor. Since the sauce thickens with refrigeration, thin it with water as needed to achieve the desired consistency.

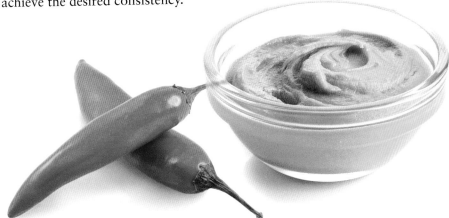

Per ⅓ cup (85 ml):
Calories: 266
Protein: 9 g
Leucine: 588 mg
Fat: 20 g
Carbohydrate: 19 g
Fiber: 3 g

Minerals:
Iron: 1.1 mg
Zinc: 1.2 mg
Calcium: 39 mg
Sodium: 368 mg

Percent of calories from:
Protein 13%
Fat 61%
Carbohydrate 26%

French Canadian PEA SOUP

This high-fiber, mineral-rich soup easily satisfies the heartiest appetites.

8 cups (2 L) low-sodium or regular vegetable broth or water, plus more as needed

2 cups (500 ml) dried green or yellow split peas, sorted and rinsed

1 large onion, diced

2 carrots, chopped

2 stalks celery, chopped

2 cloves garlic, minced

1 teaspoon (5 ml) dried thyme

1 teaspoon (5 ml) dried savory

⅛ teaspoon (0.5 ml) freshly ground black pepper

1 package (5 oz/150 g) vegan ham or bacon, chopped (optional)

Salt

Put the broth, split peas, onion, carrots, celery, garlic, thyme, savory, and pepper in a large saucepan over medium-high heat. Bring to a boil, cover, decrease the heat to medium-low, and simmer, stirring occasionally, until the peas are soft, about 1 hour.

Add the optional vegan ham and season with salt to taste. Stir to evenly distribute and warm the vegan ham. Add additional broth or water for a thinner consistency. Stored in a sealed container, the soup will keep for 5 days in the refrigerator or 6 months in the freezer.

NUTRITION NOTES: A 2-cup (500-ml) serving provides 33 grams of protein with vegan ham and 25 grams of protein without the vegan ham.

TIP: Salt is present in vegan ham, and sodium amounts vary with different broths. Taste the soup before adding any salt.

VARIATIONS: For a greater depth of flavor, add any or all of the following at the same time as the split peas: 3 bay leaves (remember to remove them before serving), ½ teaspoon (2 ml) smoked paprika, ¾ teaspoon (4 ml) ground cloves, and 1½ teaspoons (7 ml) dried marjoram. If you want to use fresh herbs, triple the amounts listed for the dried herbs.

Per 2 cups (500 ml):
Calories: 400
Protein: 25 g
Leucine: 1,670 mg
Fat: 1 g
Carbohydrate: 75 g
Fiber: 28 g

Minerals:
Iron: 5.3 mg
Zinc: 3.5 mg
Calcium: 83 mg
Sodium: 332 mg

Percent of calories from:
Protein 24%
Fat 3%
Carbohydrate 73%

Veggie Sausage and Sauerkraut SOUP

This soup is reminiscent of a traditional European soup with simple seasonings. Serve it with fresh rye bread and nut cheese to complete the meal.

1 large onion, diced

5 cups (1¼ L) low-sodium or regular vegetable broth or water

2 cups (500 ml) thinly sliced Brussels sprouts or green cabbage

2 vegan sausages (3–4 oz./90–120 g each), sliced

1 cup (250 ml) sauerkraut, drained

1 potato, chopped

1 large carrot, chopped

2 stalks celery, diced

2 tablespoons (30 ml) chopped fresh dill, or 2 teaspoons (10 ml) dried dill weed

1 tablespoon (15 ml) fresh thyme leaves, or 1 teaspoon (5 ml) dried thyme

2 cloves garlic, minced

2 bay leaves

Freshly ground black pepper

Put the onion in a large saucepan over low heat and cook, stirring constantly, until lightly browned, about 5 minutes.

Add the broth, Brussels sprouts, sausages, sauerkraut, potato, carrot, celery, dill, thyme, garlic, and bay leaves. Bring to a boil, decrease the heat to low, and simmer until all the vegetables are tender, about 45 minutes. Season with pepper to taste. Remove the bay leaves before serving. Serve hot.

VARIATION: Omit the sausages and add 1½–2 cups (375–500 ml) cooked or canned white beans (such as cannellini, great northern, or navy), drained and rinsed.

Per 2 cups (500 ml):
Calories: 238
Protein: 14 g
Leucine: 870 mg
Fat: 9 g
Carbohydrate: 30 g
Fiber: 8 g

Minerals:
Iron: 3.6 mg
Zinc: 1.3 mg
Calcium: 94 mg
Sodium: 878 mg

Percent of calories from:
Protein 22%
Fat 30%
Carbohydrate 48%

Curry IN A HURRY

Red lentils are the perfect, quick-cooking choice for this dish which also tastes great without any of the optional ingredients. Patak's Mild Curry Spice Paste is an exceptionally good seasoning choice for this thick soup, making preparation fast and easy. If you don't have access to this brand, use the Curry Paste Alternative (page 155).

4 cups (1 L) low-sodium or regular vegetable broth or water, plus more as needed

1 cup (250 ml) dried red lentils

1 onion, diced

2 tablespoons (30 ml) minced fresh ginger (optional)

4 cloves garlic, minced (optional)

1 teaspoon (5 ml) ground turmeric (optional)

2 tablespoons (30 ml) Patak's Mild Curry Spice Paste

1 can (15 oz/426 ml) stewed or crushed tomatoes (optional)

2 cups (500 ml) chopped spinach, bok choy, or kale leaves (optional)

1–2 cups (250–500 ml) cooked cauliflower, bell peppers, or carrots (optional)

½ cup (125 ml) canned coconut milk (optional)

Salt

Freshly ground black pepper

Per 1½ cups (375 ml):
Calories: 311
Protein: 18 g
Leucine 1,170
Fat: 3 g
Carbohydrate: 55 g
Fiber: 10 g

Minerals:
Iron: 6.1 mg
Zinc: 2.7 mg
Calcium: 84 mg
Sodium: 298

Percent of calories from:
Protein 23%
Fat 8%
Carbohydrate 69%

Put the broth, lentils, onion, optional ginger, optional garlic, and optional turmeric in a large saucepan. Bring to a boil over medium-high heat, decrease the heat to medium-low, and simmer until the lentils are soft, about 20 minutes. Add the curry paste, optional tomatoes, optional spinach, optional vegetables, and optional coconut milk. Stir to combine. Cook until the mixture is heated through and the greens are tender, 10–15 minutes. Season with salt and pepper to taste. Add more broth or water if a thinner consistency is desired.

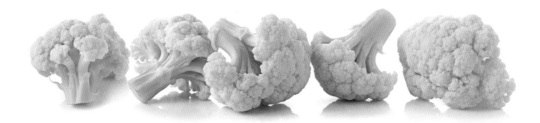

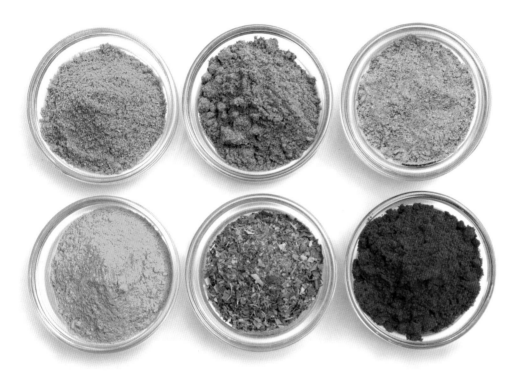

CURRY PASTE ALTERNATIVE

2 teaspoons (10 ml) curry powder

1 teaspoon (5 ml) ground turmeric

1 teaspoon (5 ml) garam masala

1 teaspoon (5 ml) ground cumin

1 teaspoon (5 ml) chili powder

½ teaspoon (2 ml) ground coriander

½ teaspoon (2 ml) salt

Put the onion that is called for in the main recipe in a large saucepan over medium heat and cook, stirring almost constantly, for 3–4 minutes. Add the spices and heat for 30–40 seconds to release their flavors. Add the water and lentils and proceed as directed in the main recipe.

VARIATIONS: Replace the red lentils with dried brown, French, gray, or green lentils, but increase the cooking time to 1 hour. In place of the cooked vegetables listed, use any leftover veggies you have on hand.

EASY-PEASY Chili

This protein-packed chili is *sin carne* (meat-free) but loaded with flavor.

CHILI

½ cup (125 ml) water or low-sodium or regular vegetable broth, plus more as needed

1 onion, chopped

1 green bell pepper, diced

2 cloves garlic, minced

28 ounces (796 ml) low-sodium or regular canned diced tomatoes, or 4 cups (1 L) chopped fresh tomatoes

1 package (10 oz./300 g) vegan burger crumbles

1½ cups (375 ml) cooked or canned kidney beans, drained and rinsed

1½ cups (375 ml) cooked or canned pinto or black beans, drained and rinsed

1 cup (250 ml) mild, medium, or hot salsa

1 teaspoon (5 ml) chili powder, plus more as needed

1 teaspoon (5 ml) dried oregano

½ teaspoon (2 ml) ground cumin

OPTIONAL TOPPINGS

Cubed avocado

Thinly sliced green onions

Chopped fresh cilantro

Shredded vegan cheese

Vegan sour cream

Lime wedges

Per 2 cups (500 ml):
Calories: 342
Protein: 27 g
Leucine: 2,194 mg
Fat: 2 g
Carbohydrate: 57 g
Fiber: 19 g

Minerals:
Iron: 11.8 mg
Zinc: 7.8 mg
Calcium: 269 mg
Sodium: 768 mg

Percent of calories from:
Protein 29%
Fat 5%
Carbohydrate 66%

Put the water, onion, bell pepper, and garlic in a large saucepan over medium-high heat and cook, stirring frequently, until the vegetables are tender, about 10 minutes. Add more water if necessary to prevent sticking. Add the tomatoes, vegan burger crumbles, kidney beans, pinto beans, salsa, chili powder, oregano, and cumin. Cook, stirring occasionally, until heated through, about 5 minutes. Cover, decrease the heat to medium-low, and simmer, stirring occasionally, until the vegetables and beans are soft and the flavors have melded, about 45 minutes.

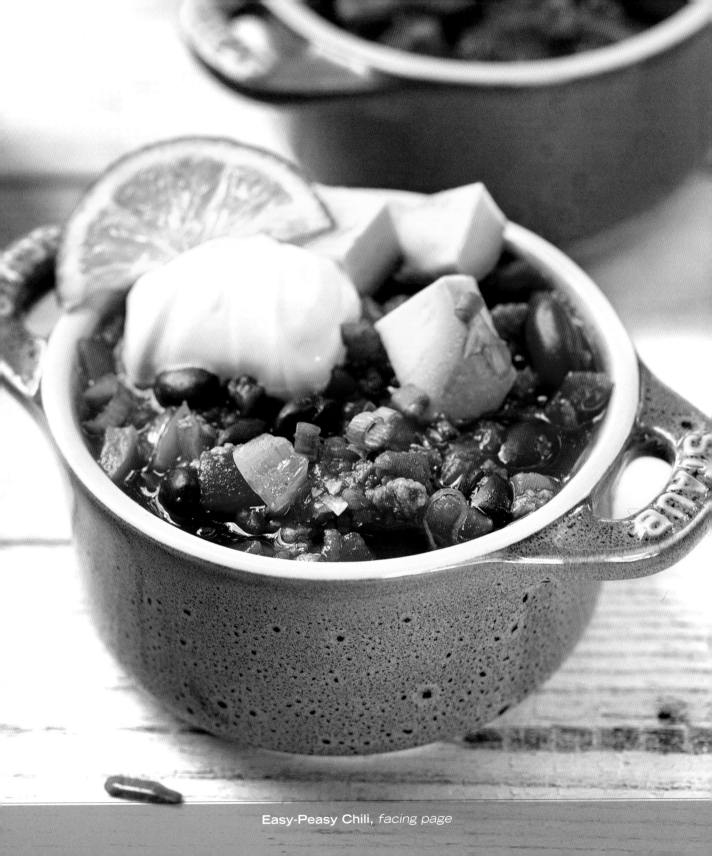

Easy-Peasy Chili, *facing page*

Add ½ cup (125 ml) water if the chili gets too dry. Serve hot with the optional toppings of your choice.

TIPS:

- If you like spice, add 1 or more finely diced hot chiles or hot sauce to taste.
- Vegan burger crumbles usually come in 10–12-ounce (300–360 g) packages. Use whatever size you purchase!
- If you prefer, replace the vegan burger crumbles with an additional 1½ cups (375 ml) cooked or canned beans.
- Boost the veggies by adding 1 cup (250 ml) frozen corn, 1 small zucchini, chopped, or 1½ cups (375 ml) cubed sweet potato at the same time as the vegan burger crumbles.

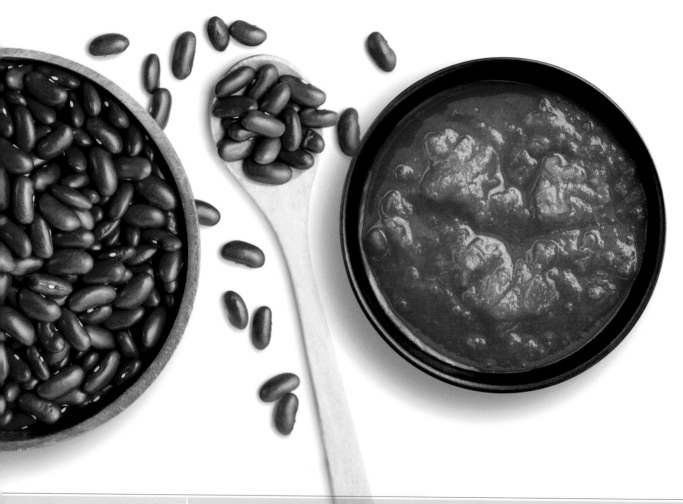

Black Bean STEW

Enjoy this protein- and mineral-rich stew with fresh rolls, bread, or crackers.

½ cup (125 ml) low-sodium or regular vegetable broth, or 1 tablespoon (15 ml) vegetable oil

1 onion, chopped

1 carrot, chopped

2 stalks celery, chopped

1 clove garlic, minced

3 cups (750 ml) low-sodium or regular vegetable broth or water

½ cup (125 ml) tomato paste

3 cups (750 ml) canned or cooked black beans, drained and rinsed

2 cups (500 ml) stemmed and thinly sliced kale, bok choy, or other greens, packed

1 tablespoon (15 ml) chopped fresh basil, or 1 teaspoon (5 ml) dried basil

1 tablespoon (15 ml) minced fresh oregano, or 1 teaspoon (5 ml) dried oregano

1 teaspoon (5 ml) ground cumin

Salt

Freshly ground black pepper

2 tablespoons (30 ml) freshly squeezed lime juice

Put the ½ cup (125 ml) of broth in a large saucepan over medium heat. Add the onion, carrot, celery, and garlic and cook, stirring occasionally, until the onion has softened, about 5 minutes.

Stir in the remaining 3 cups (750 ml) of broth and tomato paste and mix well. Add the beans, kale, basil, oregano, and cumin. Cover and simmer for 20 minutes. Season with salt and pepper to taste. Sprinkle lime juice over each serving and serve immediately. Stored in a sealed container, the stew will keep for 5 days in the refrigerator or 6 months in the freezer.

BLACK BEAN SOUP: To serve this as a soup, add vegetable broth or water to achieve the desired consistency.

VARIATIONS: For even more variety and texture, add 1 sweet potato, chopped, at the same time as the onion, or 1 cup (250 ml) corn at the same time as the beans. Add ¼ teaspoon (1 ml) cayenne or a hot chile if you enjoy a little spice.

Per 2 cups (500 ml):
Calories: 295
Protein: 18 g
Leucine: 1,200 mg
Fat: 1 g
Carbohydrate: 56 g
Fiber: 18 g

Minerals:
Iron: 5.1 mg
Zinc: 2.2 mg
Calcium: 110 mg
Sodium: 492 mg

Percent of calories from:
Protein 23%
Fat 73%
Carbohydrate 4%

STOVE-TOP Baked Beans

Classic recipes for Boston baked beans use navy beans, but you actually can use any bean you prefer or happen to have on hand. This flavorful entrée can be baked in the oven or prepared more quickly on the stove top.

1 large onion, chopped

1 cup (250 ml) water

3 cups (750 ml) cooked or canned beans, drained and rinsed

2 tablespoons (30 ml) organic blackstrap molasses or brown sugar or a mix of both

2 tablespoons (30 ml) apple cider vinegar

1 teaspoon (5 ml) Dijon mustard

1 tablespoon (15 ml) chopped fresh dill, or 1 teaspoon (5 ml) dried dill weed (optional)

½ teaspoon (2 ml) salt

¼ teaspoon (1 ml) freshly ground black pepper

¼ teaspoon (1 ml) ground cloves

2 ounces (60 g) vegan ham or bacon, chopped (optional)

Put the onion in a large, heavy saucepan over medium heat. Cook, stirring constantly, until the onion is slightly caramelized, about 5 minutes.

Put the water, beans, molasses, vinegar, mustard, optional dill, salt, pepper, cloves, and optional vegan ham in the saucepan. Mix the ingredients well, increase the heat to medium-high, and bring the mixture to a boil. Decrease the heat to medium-low and simmer, stirring occasionally, until the liquid has turned into a sauce, 30–40 minutes.

TIP: Add 2 tablespoons (30 ml) of tomato paste for a subtle umami flavor.

OVEN-BAKED BEANS: Preheat the oven to 350 degrees F (177 degrees C). Put all of the ingredients in a large casserole dish with a lid, cover, and bake for 45 minutes, stirring about every 15 minutes, until the sauce is bubbling and the onion is soft. Remove the casserole dish's lid for 15 minutes or longer to allow some of the liquid to evaporate to achieve the desired consistency, or add a little water if the beans are too dry. Baking longer (for example, 1½–2 hours) is fine, as the flavor of the dish will deepen.

Per 2 cups (500 ml):
Calories: 503
Protein: 26 g
Leucine: 2,040 mg
Fat: 2 g
Carbohydrate: 96 g
Fiber: 32 g

Minerals:
Iron: 8 mg
Zinc: 3.1 mg
Calcium: 436 mg
Sodium: 572 mg

Percent of calories from:
Protein 20%
Fat 4%
Carbohydrate 76%

Rainbow Veggie FAJITAS

Fajitas are as fun to prepare as to eat! This version provides abundant protein with vibrant colors and textures.

FAJITAS

12 ounces (360 g) firm or extra-firm tofu, cut into 2-inch x ¼-inch (5-cm x 0.6-cm) strips

2 tablespoons (30 ml) low-sodium or regular tamari

4 teaspoons (20 ml) homemade or commercial fajita seasoning mix or Tex-Mex seasoning mix (see box on page 163)

2 cups (500 ml) sliced mushrooms

1 large red onion, sliced

8 cloves garlic, thinly sliced

3 tablespoons (45 ml) low-sodium or regular vegetable broth

1 small eggplant or 1 large zucchini, cut into 2-inch x ¼-inch (5-cm x 0.6-cm) strips

1 large red bell pepper, cut into 2-inch x ¼-inch (5-cm x 0.6-cm) strips

3 cups (750 ml) chopped kale or other greens

½ cup (125 ml) chopped fresh cilantro or parsley, packed

2 tablespoons (30 ml) freshly squeezed lime juice

8 (6–7 in./15–18 cm) whole-grain or gluten-free tortillas

OPTIONAL ADDITIONS

Hot sauce	Sliced avocado	Vegan sour cream
Hot chiles	Shredded vegan cheese	Lime wedges
Guacamole		

Per 2 fajitas:
Calories: 333
Protein: 18 g
Leucine: 1,086 mg
Fat: 9 g
Carbohydrate: 48 g
Fiber: 7 g

Minerals:
Iron: 5.4 mg
Zinc: 1.8 mg
Calcium: 337 mg
Sodium: 861 mg*

Percent of calories from:
Protein 21%
Fat 24%
Carbohydrate 55%

*Sodium per serving can vary from 672 to 1,251 milligrams depending on your choice of ingredients.

Preheat the oven to 350 degrees F (177 degrees C). Line a large baking sheet with a silicone baking mat or parchment paper, or mist the baking sheet with cooking spray. Arrange the tofu on the prepared baking sheet and brush the tofu with 1 tablespoon (15 ml) of the tamari and sprinkle it with 2 teaspoons (10 ml) of the fajita seasoning mix. Bake for 20 minutes, or until the tofu is slightly crispy.

Put the mushrooms in a large skillet or nonstick pan over medium heat and cook, stirring constantly, until lightly browned, about 5 minutes. Add the onion, garlic, and vegetable broth and cook, stirring frequently, for 5 minutes.

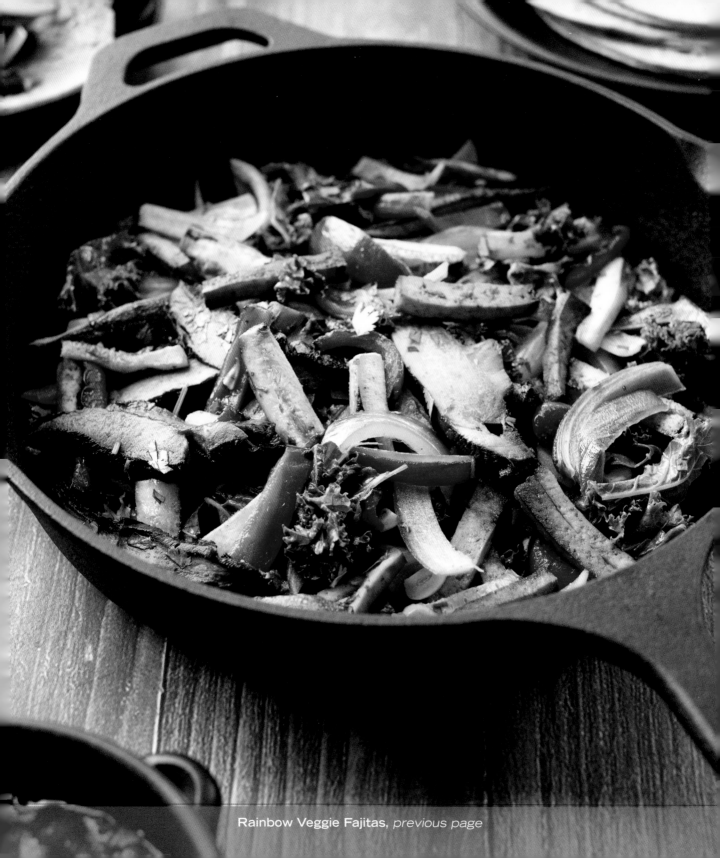

Rainbow Veggie Fajitas, *previous page*

Add the eggplant, bell pepper, remaining 1 tablespoon (15 ml) of tamari, and remaining 2 teaspoons (10 ml) of fajita seasoning mix. Cook, stirring frequently, until the eggplant is tender, about 10 minutes. Add the kale and cook, stirring frequently, for 3 minutes. Gently stir in the tofu, cilantro, and lime juice.

Assemble the fajitas by placing ¾ cup (185 ml) of the fajita mixture lengthwise in the center of the tortillas. Top with the optional additions of your choice. Squeeze optional lime wedges generously over the filling. Fold each side of the tortillas toward the filling and serve.

TIP: Feel free to use seasoned tofu (or any other plant-based protein alternatives).

HOMEMADE FAJITA SEASONING

2 teaspoons (10 ml) chili powder

½ teaspoon (2 ml) ground cumin

½ teaspoon (2 ml) smoked paprika

½ teaspoon (2 ml) garlic powder

½ teaspoon (2 ml) onion powder

Put all the ingredients in a small jar, seal tightly, and shake well to thoroughly combine.

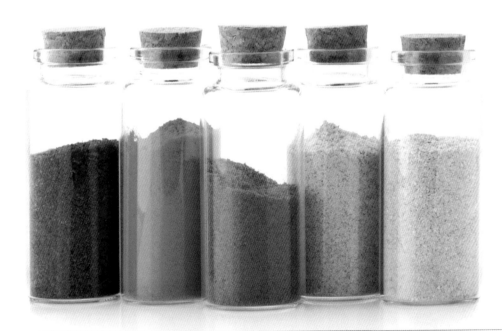

The Big Bowl

Dinner bowls are fast, easy, and satisfying, and this one is particularly high in protein and minerals. Replace the vegetables with your personal favorites or increase the quantity of vegetables called for in the ingredients.

BOWL

1½ cups (375 ml) quartered Brussels sprouts

1 carrot, cut in half lengthwise and thinly sliced on the diagonal

1 cup (250 ml) cauliflower florets

½ red bell pepper, thinly sliced

2 cups stemmed and chopped kale or other leafy greens, packed

2 cups (500 ml) cooked whole grains (such as barley, black rice, farro, Kamut, or quinoa)

1½ cups (375 ml) cooked or canned beans (such as black beans, chickpeas, edamame, or kidney beans), drained and rinsed

Ginger, Lime, and Miso Dressing (page 150) or other dressing of choice

OPTIONAL ADDITIONS

Sliced avocado

Peanuts

Toasted sesame, sunflower, or pumpkin seeds

Toasted almonds

Sprouts

Sliced green onions

Chopped or torn fresh herbs (such as basil, cilantro, or parsley)

Hot sauce

Per one-half recipe*:
Calories: 457
Protein: 28 g
Leucine 1,018 mg
Fat: 11 g
Carbohydrate: 68 g
Fiber: 18 g

Minerals:
Iron: 7.4 mg
Zinc: 4.5 mg
Calcium: 190 mg
Sodium: 84 mg

Percent of calories from:
Protein 23%
Fat 20%
Carbohydrate 57%

*The analysis was done without the Ginger, Lime, and Miso Dressing (see page 150 for analysis of the dressing).

Put the Brussels sprouts and carrot in a large saucepan fitted with a large steamer basket. Fill the saucepan about one-quarter full with water (the water shouldn't touch the steamer basket). Bring the water to a simmer over medium heat. Cover and steam the vegetables for 4 minutes. Add the cauliflower and bell pepper and steam for 4 minutes. Add the kale and steam for 2 minutes.

Assemble the dinner bowls by putting 1 cup (250 ml) of the cooked grains at the base of each bowl. Add the steamed vegetables and beans, using half the vegetables and beans for each bowl. Top each serving with the Ginger, Lime, and Miso Dressing, or pass the dressing at the table.

VARIATIONS: Swap out the beans for seasoned tofu or tempeh or vegan beef or vegan chicken. Asparagus, cabbage, green beans, onions, snow peas, or squash would make excellent additions to this bowl.

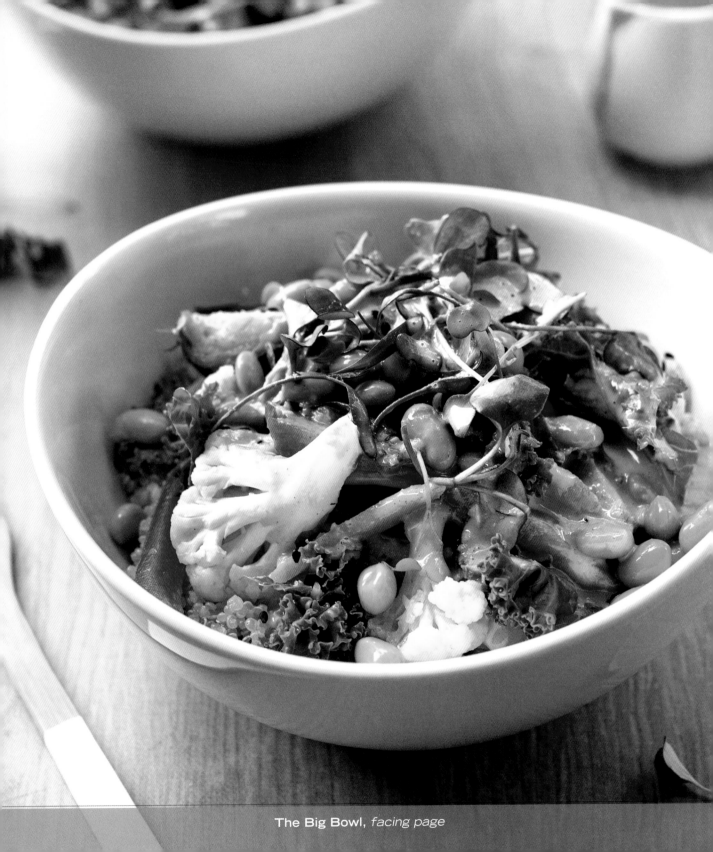

The Big Bowl, *facing page*

HEARTY Vegetable Dahl

This dahl can be made with any vegetables you have on hand. Serve it with brown rice, naan, or popadam.

1½ teaspoons (7 ml) cumin seeds

1 onion, chopped

3 cloves garlic, minced

1½ tablespoons (22 ml) minced or grated fresh ginger

5 cups (1.25 L) low-sodium or regular vegetable broth or water

1½ cups (375 ml) split yellow mung beans or red lentils

2 carrots, cut in half lengthwise and chopped diagonally in ½-inch (1.5-cm) pieces

1½ teaspoons (7 ml) garam masala or curry powder

1 teaspoon (5 ml) ground turmeric

1½ cups (375 ml) cauliflower florets

1½ cups (375 ml) broccoli florets

1 red bell pepper, chopped, or 2 tomatoes, chopped

2 cups (500 ml) stemmed and chopped kale, spinach, or other dark greens, packed

¾ cup (185 ml) fortified unsweetened coconut milk, cashew cream, or canned coconut milk

Salt

Freshly ground black pepper

Lime or lemon wedges

Per 2 cups (500 ml):
Calories: 336
Protein: 21 g
Leucine: 1,498 mg
Fat: 2 g
Carbohydrate: 61 g
Fiber: 16 g

Minerals:
Iron: 6.7 mg
Zinc: 2.5 mg
Calcium: 217 mg
Sodium: 846 mg

Percent of calories from:
Protein 24%
Fat 6%
Carbohydrate 70%

*Analysis was done with fortified unsweetened coconut milk.

Put the cumin seeds in a large saucepan over medium-low heat and cook, stirring constantly, for 1 minute. Add the onion, garlic, ginger, and ½ cup (125 ml) of the broth. Cook, stirring frequently, until the onion is soft, about 5 minutes.

Add the remaining 4½ cups (1.1 L) of the broth, mung beans, carrots, garam masala, and turmeric. Increase the heat to high. Bring the mixture to a boil, stir, cover the saucepan, and decrease the heat to low. Simmer, stirring occasionally, until the beans are soft, 30–40 minutes. Add the cauliflower, broccoli, and bell pepper and cook, stirring occasionally, for 10 minutes. Remove the saucepan from the heat and stir in the kale and coconut milk. Cover and let rest for 5–10 minutes to wilt the kale. Season to taste with salt and pepper. Serve with lime wedges.

TIP: Toasting cumin seeds briefly in a pan helps intensify their flavor.

Creamy Mushroom-Broccoli SAUCE

MAKES 7 CUPS (1.75 L)

This creamy pasta sauce uses cashews to replace butter and cream. Swap the broccoli or broccolini for a combination of cauliflower and chopped greens (such as collards, kale, or spinach) or bite-size pieces of asparagus. Serve the sauce with legume pasta (such as chickpea, edamame, or lentil) for a potent protein boost. Top each serving with grated vegan cheese for an authentic flavor boost!

3 cups (750 ml) fortified unsweetened soy milk or other nondairy milk

¾ cup (175 ml) raw cashews, soaked 2–4 hours and drained

2 tablespoons (30 ml) nutritional yeast flakes

2 tablespoons (30 ml) cornstarch

2 tablespoons (30 ml) freshly squeezed lemon juice

1 teaspoon (5 ml) salt

3 cups (750 ml) sliced mushrooms

1 white onion, chopped

6 cloves garlic, minced

½ cup (125 ml) low-sodium or regular vegetable broth

3 cups (750 ml) broccoli florets or chopped broccolini

2 cups (500 ml) frozen green peas

1 red bell pepper, sliced into thin strips

¼ cup (60 ml) chopped fresh basil or parsley, lightly packed

Freshly ground black pepper

Per 1¾ cups (438 ml)*:
Calories: 382
Protein: 21 g
Leucine 1,110 mg
Fat: 15 g
Carbohydrate: 46 g
Fiber: 9 g

Minerals:
Iron: 5.6 mg
Zinc: 3.3 mg
Calcium: 131 mg
Sodium: 798 mg

Percent of calories from:
Protein 20%
Fat 34%
Carbohydrate 46%

*The analysis was done without the pasta or cheese mentioned in the headnote.

Put the milk, cashews, nutritional yeast flakes, cornstarch, lemon juice, and salt in a blender and process on high speed until silky smooth.

Put the mushrooms in a large skillet over medium-low heat and cook, stirring constantly, for 5 minutes. Add the onion and garlic, and cook, stirring constantly, for 5 minutes. Stir in the broth, decrease the heat to low, and cook, stirring occasionally, for 3 minutes. Add the broccoli, peas, and bell pepper, cover, and cook for 5 minutes.

Pour the cashew milk mixture into the skillet and cook, stirring constantly, until the mixture thickens, 2–3 minutes. Add the basil and season with pepper to taste.

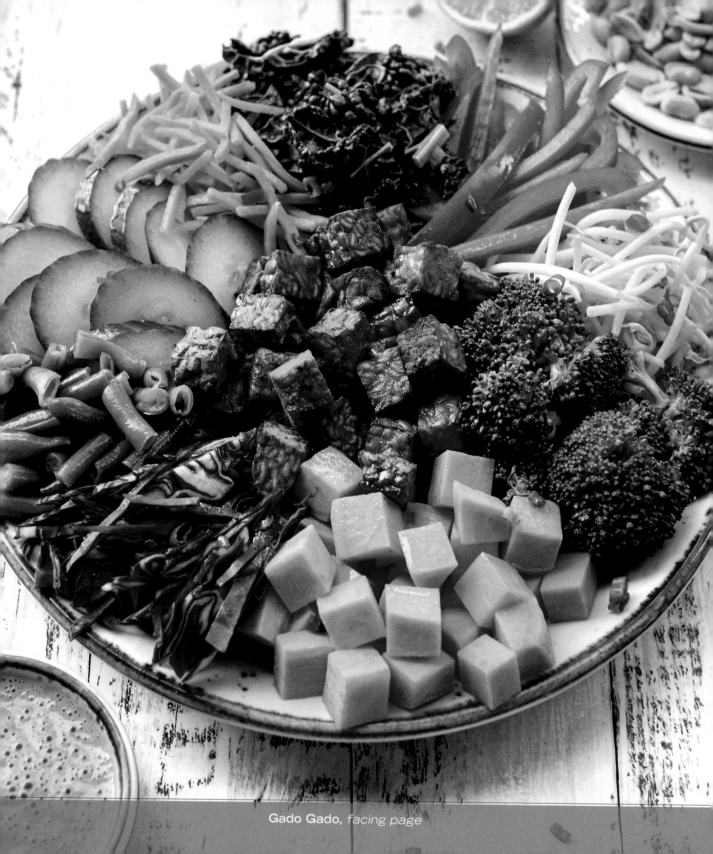

Gado Gado, *facing page*

Gado Gado

Gado gado is one of Indonesia's five national dishes. It consists of vegetables that are raw or steamed until crisp-tender, plus tofu or tempeh. Then it's topped with a spicy peanut sauce. We give the dish a healthy lift by baking rather than frying the tofu or tempeh and omitting the oil in the sauce. Get creative with the vegetables and include local and seasonal choices.

TOFU OR TEMPEH

12 ounces (360 g) firm tofu or tempeh, cut into ¾-inch (2-cm) cubes

1 tablespoon (15 ml) low-sodium or regular tamari

1 teaspoon (5 ml) salt-free seasoning blend of choice

½ teaspoon (2 ml) ground turmeric

VEGETABLES

2 sweet potatoes, peeled and cubed

2 cups (500 ml) cut green beans

2 cups (500 ml) broccoli florets and pieces

4 cups (1 L) chopped leafy greens (such as bok choy, kale, or collards)

2 cups (500 ml) mung bean sprouts

2 cups (500 ml) finely shredded red cabbage

2 carrots, shredded

1 cucumber, thinly sliced

1 red bell pepper, sliced into strips

OPTIONAL TOPPINGS

½ cup (125 ml) sliced green onions

½ cup (125 ml) chopped fresh cilantro, lightly packed

¼ cup (60 ml) crushed unsalted dry-roasted peanuts

Lime wedges

Hot sauce

Gado Gado Sauce (page 151), for serving

Per serving (one-fourth recipe)*:
Calories: 235
Protein: 16 g
Leucine: 1,018 mg
Fat: 5 g
Carbohydrate: 39 g
Fiber: 10 g

Minerals:
Iron: 4.9 mg
Zinc: 2 mg
Calcium: 371 mg
Sodium: 406 mg

Percent of calories from:
Protein 25%
Fat 16%
Carbohydrate 59%

*The analysis was done without the Gado Gado Sauce (see page 151 for analysis of the sauce).

To make the tofu or tempeh, preheat the oven to 350 degrees F (177 degrees C). Line a medium baking sheet with a silicone baking mat or parchment paper. Put the tofu or tempeh in a medium bowl. Coat with the tamari, seasoning blend, and turmeric. Transfer the tofu or tempeh to the prepared baking sheet. Bake the tofu or tempeh for 20 minutes, or until crispy. Transfer it to a medium bowl.

Steam the vegetables in two batches. Start by steaming the sweet potatoes for 2 minutes. Add the green beans and steam for 2 minutes. Add the broccoli and steam for 4 minutes. Arrange the sweet potatoes, green beans, and broccoli on a large platter or on individual plates.

Steam the leafy greens for 2 minutes. Add the bean sprouts and steam for 1 minute. Arrange the leafy greens, bean sprouts, cabbage, carrots, cucumber, bell pepper, and tofu or tempeh on the platter. Serve with the optional toppings of your choice. Top with Gado Gado Sauce, or pass the sauce at the table.

ACKNOWLEDGMENTS

We would like to thank Book Publishing Company, which has helped us bring forth 13 books over the past three decades and which are now in nine languages. It has been a delight to work with our editor, Lorne Mallin, who has taken such care at every step, and with our managing and recipe editor, Jo Stepaniak. We are indebted to the entire Book Publishing team, particularly Bob Holzapfel, Anna Pope, and Michael Thomas, for their expertise, energy, and encouragement. Special thanks to Hannah Kaminsky for her beautiful food photography.

We will be forever grateful to our skilled recipe testers and dear friends Liliana Cruz Vallejo, Lynn Isted, Margie Colclough, and Daneen Agecoutay, who spent many hours and many weeks testing recipes to ensure that they would be delicious as well as foolproof and easy to follow. We are deeply grateful for all the care and attention you gave to testing the recipes and for your invaluable feedback and creative suggestions. Many thanks to Dilip Barman for his Hearty Vegetable Dahl and ongoing encouragement, and to Donelda Rose for her marinade recipe used with the Tasty Tofu Fingers. With appreciation as well to Andres Vallejo, Art Isted, and Stacey Agecoutay, who served as brilliant food critics. Thanks to Joseph Forest, coauthor of *Cooking Vegan*, for his earlier work on the Full of Beans Salad, Kale Salad with Orange-Ginger Dressing, French Canadian Pea Soup, Black Bean Stew, and Stove-Top Baked Beans.

With appreciation to Elena Kwan for retrieving research articles for us and doing so in such a kind and timely manner, and to Dr. Matthew Nagra for his support and understanding of plant protein. We also thank ESHA Research (esha.com) for their outstanding nutritional analysis program, the Food Processor.

Finally, we would like to thank our dear spouses, Paul Davis, Cam Doré, and Josie Jiang, and our families, who have never failed to provide support, inspiration, and love throughout the process.

ABOUT THE AUTHORS

Brenda Davis, RD, is one of the world's leading plant-based pioneers and an internationally acclaimed speaker. Widely regarded as a rock star of plant-based nutrition, she has been referred to by *VegNews* as the "godmother" of vegan dietitians and was the 2022 recipient of the Plantrician Project's Luminary Award. Brenda's work focuses on ensuring that everyone who wishes to be plant-based can succeed brilliantly. She lives in Alberta, Canada, with her husband, Paul. Visit her at brendadavisrd.com.

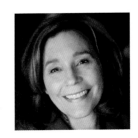

Vesanto Melina, MS, RD, is a sought-after speaker at health conferences worldwide. A consultant for individuals as well as the government of British Columbia, she is the lead author of the last position paper on vegetarian diets for the Academy of Nutrition and Dietetics. Also, Vesanto received the prestigious Ryley-Jeffs Memorial Award from Dietitians of Canada. She resides in Vancouver, Canada, with her partner, Cam. Her website is nutrispeak.com.

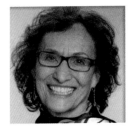

Cory Davis, MBA, P.Ag, is a professional agrologist who has worked in natural resource management since 2012 and has been a lifelong advocate for animal welfare and environmental stewardship. His broad range of experience and diverse degrees encompassing business, the sciences, and intercultural relations have given him a unique, integrated perspective on sustainable practices and their effects on human health and well-being. Cory lives in British Columbia, Canada.

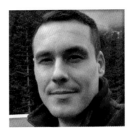

INDEX

A

Academy of Nutrition and Dietetics, 21, 87, 88t, 89

Acid reflux, 9

Adequate intake (AI), of protein for infants, 73–74

Adventist Health Study, 16, 27, 54, 99

Adventist Health Study-2 (AHS-2), 16, 54

Adzuki beans, 23, 32t

Agricultural Adjustment Act (1933), 3

Agriculture. *See also* Animal agriculture
    farm subsidies and, 3–4, 43
    land use for, 43–45
    subsidies, 3–4, 43
    water consumption and, 46
    water pollution and, 48–49

Agriculture Fairness Alliance, 3

ALA (alpha-linolenic acid), 101

Alanine, 21

Allergies, 85

Almond butter, 23, 33t. *See also* Nut butters

Almond milk
    added sugar in vanilla, 76
    calories, protein, and the percentage of calories from protein, carbohydrates, and fat in, 38t
    nutrition in, 77t

Almonds, 61. *See also* Nuts

calories, protein, and the percentage of calories from protein, carbohydrates, and fat in, 33t

Powered-Up Overnight Oats, 125

protein, leucine, and lysine in, 24t

Aluminum, in soy formula, 77

Alzheimer's disease, 60t

Amaranth
    calories, protein, and the percentage of calories from protein, carbohydrates, and fat in, 34t
    cooking time, 122t
    essential amino acids in, 19
    protein in, 107
    protein, leucine, and lysine in, 25t

American Academy of Pediatrics, 77

American College of Sports Medicine, 87, 88t, 89

American Institute of Cancer Research, 56

Amino acids. *See also* Branched-chain amino acids
    about, 19
    for athletes, 88t
    branched-chain, 22–23, 22–26, 22f
    "conditionally essential," 20–21
    estimating daily requirements of, 21
    insulin, 8
    in life cycle of a protein, 9–10
    needs during pregnancy and lactation, 71

nine essential, 10, 19–20

protein quality assessment tool and, 2

protein synthesis and, 10, 21

rating protein quality and, 2

sequence of insulin, 8

supplements, 9, 21–22, 92–93

synthesized from other amino acids, 21

Animal agriculture
    climate change and, 41
    environmental harm and, 49–50
    land use and, 43–45
    water pollution and, 49

Animal feed
    corn and, 48
    GMO plantations for, 47
    land use and, 43, 44
    soybean production and, 46, 47, 48

Animal fodder, 2, 3, 44

Animal products
    belief on "real" source of protein from, 1
    calories, protein, and the percentage of calories from protein, carbohydrates, and fat in, 39t
    percentage of protein from, 16
    policies encouraging, 2
    protein quality assessment tool and, 2
    thought of as protein foods, 31

Animal protein
  athletes swapping plant-based
    protein for, 86–87
  benefits of plant-based protein
    over, 90
  comparing plant-based protein
    to, 16
  global supply, 63t, 64
  health impact of plant protein
    versus, 51–53, 58–59, 59–60t
  overestimation of protein quality
    with, 2
  plant protein replacing as we age,
    99
Antioxidants, 59t
Apples, 37t
Apricots, 37t
Apricots (dried), 37t
Arginine, 20
Artificial sweeteners, 20
Arugula, 35t
Asparagine, 21
Asparagus
  amino acids and, 23
  calories, protein, and the percent-
    age of calories from protein,
    carbohydrates, and fat in, 35t
Aspartame, 20
Aspartate, 21
Aspartic acid, 20
Assisted living facilities, 100
Athletes, 86–94
  advantages of plant protein for,
    90
  branched-chain amino acids for,
    88–89
  comparison of animal-based
    and plant-based diets for, 16
  getting too much protein, 94
  menu ideas for, 109t
  with plant-based diets, 5
  protein boosts for, 91, 91t
  protein needs, 13, 87–88, 88t

protein powders for, 93–94
recommended protein intake
  for, 87–88, 88t, 108t
story of Sonya Looney, 86–87
sufficiency of protein for building muscle mass in, 89
supplements for, 92–93
timing of protein intake for, 89
Australia
  daily protein supply in, 63t, 64
  elimination of farm subsidies in, 4
Avocados
  amino acids and, 23
  calories, protein, and the per-
    centage of calories from pro-
    tein, carbohydrates, and fat
    in, 35t
  prepping, 119
  as source of fat, 104
  used instead of oils in dressings,
    116
Awesome Burger, 32t

B

Banana
  calories, protein, and the per-
    centage of calories from pro-
    tein, carbohydrates, and fat
    in, 37t
  Gorilla Granola, 127–128
  in Green Power Smoothie, 124
Barley. *See also* Whole grains
  calories, protein, and the per-
    centage of calories from pro-
    tein, carbohydrates, and fat
    in, 34t
  cooking times for, 122t
  greenhouse gas emissions and,
    42f
  land use and, 45f
  water consumption and, 47f
  water pollution and, 49f

Bean dishes, getting your
  child(ren) to like, 84–85
Bean pasta, 61
Beans. *See also* specific beans
  The Big Bowl, 164
  Black Bean Stew, 159
  cooking, 119–120
  Easy-Peasy Chili, 156–158
  essential amino acids in, 19
  Full of Beans Salad, 141
  Power Greens Salad, 138
  presoaking, 118, 119–120
  Stove-Top Baked Beans, 160
  in your pantry, 112
Beans (snap green/yellow), 35t
*Becoming Vegan: Comprehensive
  Edition* (Davis and Melina),
  86
Beef
  calories, protein, and the percent-
    age of calories from protein,
    carbohydrates, and fat in, 39t
  greenhouse gas emissions and,
    42, 42f
  land use and, 44, 45f
  water consumption and, 46, 47f
  water pollution and, 48–49, 49f
Beet greens, 35t
Beetroot juice, 35t
Beets, 35t
Bell peppers. *See* Peppers (bell)
Beta-alanine, 87, 92
Beyond Burgers, 29, 30, 32t
Beyond Sausage, 33t
The Big Bowl, 164
Biological Value, 2
Black beans
  Black Bean Stew, 159
  calories, protein, and the percent-
    age of calories from protein,
    carbohydrates, and fat in, 32t
  Double-Chocolate Surprise
    Cookies, 135

Easy-Peasy Chili, 156
Black Bean Stew, 159
Blackberries, 37t
Black-eyed peas, 32t
Blackstrap molasses, 114, 115
  Stove-Top Baked Beans, 160
Black walnuts, 61
Blueberries, 37t
BMI, estimating your, 71
Body weight, protein needs during
    pregnancy and, 71, 71t
Bok choy, 35t. *See also* Leafy greens
Bone strength/health, 16, 96
Bragg Liquid Aminos, 114, 133,
    143, 144
Branched-chain amino acids. *See
    also* Leucine
  for athletes, 88–89, 88t
  foods with, 23, 24–25t
  functions of, 19–20, 22, 88–89
  supplements, 9, 25–26, 93, 99
Brazil
  daily protein supply in, 63t
  dietary guidelines, 66
  livestock-driven deforestation
    in, 43
Brazil nuts. *See also* Nuts
  calories, protein, and the percent-
    age of calories from protein,
    carbohydrates, and fat in, 33t
  protein, leucine, and lysine in, 24t
Bread, 34t
Breakfast
  adding protein to, for muscle
    building, 82
  examples of simple protein
    boosts for, 91t
  menu ideas, 108t
Breastfeeding, 72–73. *See also*
    Lactation
Breast milk, 72, 73–74
Broccoli florets
  amino acids and, 23

calories, protein, and the percent-
    age of calories from protein,
    carbohydrates, and fat in, 35t
  Creamy Mushroom-Broccoli
    Sauce, 167
  Gado Gado, 169–170
  Hearty Vegetable Dahl, 166
Brown rice
  calories, protein, and the percent-
    age of calories from protein,
    carbohydrates, and fat in, 35t
  cooking time, 122t
  protein, leucine, and lysine in, 25t
Brussels sprouts
  The Big Bowl, 164
  calories, protein, and the percent-
    age of calories from protein,
    carbohydrates, and fat in, 35t
  Veggie Sausage and Sauerkraut
    Soup, 153
Buckwheat. *See also* Whole grains
  cooking time, 122t
  essential amino acids in, 19
  protein, leucine, and lysine in, 25t
Buckwheat groats, 34t
Bulgur, 122t

C

Cabbage
  calories, protein, and the percent-
    age of calories from protein,
    carbohydrates, and fat in, 35t
  Gado Gado, 169–170
  Kale Salad with Orange-Ginger
    Dressing, 143
  Peanut-Edamame Noodle Salad,
    144
  Power Greens Salad, 138
  Veggie Sausage and Sauerkraut
    Soup, 153
Calcium
  for bone health, 96

in different types of milk, 77t
in fortified milks, 76, 105
high protein intakes and, 96
low intakes among vegan youth,
    81
milks fortified with, 105
sources of, in fruits, 103t
sources of, in legumes, 103t
sources of, in vegetables, 103t
soy milk and, 98
Calories
  in animal products, 39t
  calculating protein as percent
    of, 15
  in different types of milk, 77t
  in fruits, 37–38t
  in grains, 34–35t
  in legumes and, 32–33t
  from macronutrients, 7
  in nondairy beverages, 38t
  in nuts and seeds, 33–34t
  in oils, fats, and sweeteners, 38t
  plant foods delivering fewer, 90
  protein as a percent of, 15
  in vegetables, 35–37t
Cambodia, daily protein supply in,
    63t, 64
Canada
  daily protein supply in, 63t, 64
  dietary guidelines and food
    guide, 67
  Health Canada, 67
  subsidies in, 3–4
Cancers
  high protein intake and, 96
  methionine and, 20
  protein sources and, 56–58
  red meat and, 16
  soy and, 26, 27, 77
Canderel, 20
Cantaloupe, 37t
Carbohydrates
  about, 7

animal products lacking, 31
cardiovascular disease and, 53
glycogen stores and, 90
in natural plant foods, 31
percent of calories in typical serv-
    ings of various foods, 32–39t
Carbon, 7, 8
Carboxypeptidase, 9
Cardiovascular disease. *See* Heart
    health
Cargill, 5
Carnosine, 92
Carrot juice, 35t
Carrots
    calories, protein, and the percent-
        age of calories from protein,
        carbohydrates, and fat in, 35t
    Carrot Spice Cookies, 137
    Curry in a Hurry, 154
    French Canadian Pea Soup, 152
    Gado Gado, 169–170
    Hearty Vegetable Dahl, 166
    Peanut-Edamame Noodle Salad,
        144
    as protein booster in Green
        Power Smoothie, 124
    Veggie Sausage and Sauerkraut
        Soup, 153
Carrot Spice Cookies, 106, 137
Cashew butter, 33t. *See also* Nut
    butters
Cashew milk, 77t
Cashews
    as base for dairy replacements,
        85
    calories, protein, and the per-
        centage of calories from pro-
        tein, carbohydrates, and fat
        in, 33t
    Creamy Mushroom-Broccoli
        Sauce, 167
    protein, leucine, and lysine in, 24t
    in your pantry, 112

Cattle, land use and, 44
Cauliflower
    The Big Bowl, 164
    calories, protein, and the percent-
        age of calories from protein,
        carbohydrates, and fat in, 35t
    Curry in a Hurry, 154
    Hearty Vegetable Dahl, 166
Celery
    Black Bean Stew, 159
    calories, protein, and the percent-
        age of calories from protein,
        carbohydrates, and fat in, 35t
    French Canadian Pea Soup, 152
    as protein booster in Green
        Power Smoothie, 124
    Tangy Chickpea Smash, 147
    Veggie Sausage and Sauerkraut
        Soup, 153
Cheese
    calories, protein, and the per-
        centage of calories from pro-
        tein, carbohydrates, and fat in
        cheddar, 39t
    fresh water consumption and,
        46, 47f
    greenhouse gas emissions and,
        42f
    land use and, 45f
    vegan, 113
    water consumption and, 46, 47f
    water pollution and, 49f
Chemical contaminants, 60t
Cherries, 37t
Chia Pudding, 98, 134
Chia seeds
    calories, protein, and the percent-
        age of calories from protein,
        carbohydrates, and fat in, 33t
    Gorilla Granola, 127–128
    omega-3 fatty acids in, 101, 112
    Powered-Up Overnight Oats, 125
    protein, leucine, and lysine in, 24t

    Vanilla Chia Pudding, 134
Chicken breast, 39t
Chickpeas (garbanzo). *See also*
    Beans
    calories, protein, and the percent-
        age of calories from protein,
        carbohydrates, and fat in, 32t
    Power Greens Salad, 138
    Tangy Chickpea Smash, 147
Children and teens
    fitting in with friends on a plant-
        based diet, 83–84
    long-term consequences of
        plant-protein diet for, 81–82
    menu ideas for, 109t
    muscle-making on plant-based
        diet, 82–83
    on a plant-based diet, 79
    protein needs, 13, 80–81, 81t
    recommended protein intake, 108
    serving sizes for, 101
Chili. *See* Easy-Peasy Chili
China
    cancer and protein sources in,
        58
    cardiovascular disease and pro-
        tein sources in, 53–54
    daily protein supply in, 63t, 64
    dietary guidelines, 68
    mortality and protein sources
        in, 52
    type 2 diabetes and protein
        sources in, 55
Chocolate Chia Pudding, 134
Chocolate chunks/chips, in Double-
    Chocolate Surprise Cookies,
    135
Cholesterol
    health effects, 60t
    lowering LDL, 27
    meat alternatives and, 29
    in plant versus animal protein,
        60t

Chronic disease(s)
    cancer, 56–58
    heart disease, 3–4, 53–55
    lifestyle choices and, 95
    plant protein reducing risk of, 99
    recommended protein and leucine
        intakes for people with, 98–99
    type 2 diabetes, 55–56
Chymotrypsin, 9
Circulation, plant-protein foods
    improving, 90
Climate Change and Land (IPCC),
    66
Climate change/crisis. *See also*
    Environmental issues; Green-
    house gas emissions
    animal agriculture and, 41
    attraction of plant-based diet
        and, 28
    dietary shift and, 50
    economic costs, 40–41
    extreme weather events and, 40
    increase in average global tem-
        perature, 40
    IPCC Special Report on, 66
    land use and, 43–45
    political and social repercus-
        sions of, 42–43
    and shifting subsidies to veg-
        etables and fruits, 4
Coconut (dried)
    calories, protein, and the percent-
        age of calories from protein,
        carbohydrates, and fat in, 37t
    Gorilla Granola, 127–128
Coconut milk
    compared with other milks, 77t
    Curry in a Hurry, 154
    Ginger, Lime, and Miso Dress-
        ing, 150
    Hearty Vegetable Dahl, 166
Collard greens
    amino acids and, 23

calories, protein, and the percent-
    age of calories from protein,
    carbohydrates, and fat in, 35t
    Power Greens Salad, 138
Colombia, daily protein supply in,
    63t
Colon, protein overconsumption
    and, 16
Colorectal cancer, 56
Complete protein, 10–11
Condiments, 114
Cookies
    Carrot Spice Cookies, 137
    Double-Chocolate Surprise
        Cookies, 135
Corn
    amino acids and, 23
    for animal feed, 48
    calories, protein, and the percent-
        age of calories from protein,
        carbohydrates, and fat in, 36t
    farm subsidies for, 3
    Full of Beans Salad, 141
    greenhouse gas emissions and, 42f
    land use and, 45f
    protein, leucine, and lysine in, 25t
    water consumption and, 47f
    water pollution and, 49f
Cornmeal, 34t
Corn protein, in protein powders, 93
Corn tortilla, 34t
Cow's milk, 31
    calories, protein, and the percent-
        age of calories from protein,
        carbohydrates, and fat in, 39t
    in early North America, 4
    nutrition in, 77t
Cranberries, 37t
Cranberry beans, 32t
Creamy Mushroom-Broccoli Sauce,
    167
Creamy Vanilla Chai Pudding, 106,
    134

Creatine, 22, 92–93
Cropland, 44
Cucumber
    calories, protein, and the percent-
        age of calories from protein,
        carbohydrates, and fat in, 36t
    food prep and, 119
    Gado Gado, 169–170
    Lentil Tabbouleh, 142
Currants (dried)
    calories, protein, and the percent-
        age of calories from protein,
        carbohydrates, and fat in, 37t
    Gorilla Granola, 127–128
Curry in a Hurry, 105, 154–155
Cysteine, 2, 8, 20

D
Dahl, Hearty Vegetable, 166
Dairy cattle, 44, 46, 48
Dairy farms
    Canadian, 4
    farm subsidies for, 2, 3, 4
Dates
    calories, protein, and the percent-
        age of calories from protein,
        carbohydrates, and fat in, 37t
    Carrot Spice Cookies, 137
    Double-Chocolate Surprise
        Cookies, 135
    Gado Gado Sauce, 151
    Gorilla Granola, 127–128
    Orange-Ginger Dressing, 143
    Vanilla Chia Pudding, 134
Davis, Brenda, 86
Davis, Cory, 41
Deforestation, 43–45, 49
Deli slices, vegan, 83, 98, 106
    calories, protein, and the percent-
        age of calories from protein,
        carbohydrates, and fat in, 33t
Dementia, 99, 100

Denmark, daily protein supply in, 63t
Desertification, 49
DHA (docosahexaenoic acid), 101
DIAAS (Digestible Indispensable Amino Acid Score), 11, 12
Dietitians of Canada, 87, 88t, 89
Digestibility
   food preparation and, 13
   of protein, 11–12
Dinner
   examples of simple protein boosts for, 91t
   incorporating protein into, for muscle building, 83
   menu ideas, 108t
   for seniors, 98
DNA, 10
Double-Chocolate Surprise Cookies, 109t, 135
Dressings
   avoiding oil in, 116
   Ginger, Lime, and Miso Dressing, 150
   Hummus and Lime Dressing, 149
   Lemon-Tahini Protein-Plus Dressing, 148
   Orange-Ginger Dressing, 143
   Peanut Dressing, 144
Dried fruit(s), 113, 115, 125. See also Dates; Raisins
Droughts, 45
Dry sautéing, 115
Dulse flakes, 147
Durian, 37t

E

Easy-Peasy Chili, 105, 109t, 156–158
EAT-Lancet Commission on Food, Planet, Health, 65

Edamame, 23, 27, 85, 112
   calories, protein, and the percentage of calories from protein, carbohydrates, and fat in, 32t
   Peanut-Edamame Noodle Salad, 144
   Power Greens Salad, 138
   protein, leucine, and lysine in, 24t
Edema, 15
Eggplant
   calories, protein, and the percentage of calories from protein, carbohydrates, and fat in, 36t
   Rainbow Veggie Fajitas, 161–163
Eggs
   calories, protein, and the percentage of calories from protein, carbohydrates, and fat in, 39t
   greenhouse gas emissions and, 42f
   land use and, 45f
   water consumption and, 47f
   water pollution and, 49f
Egypt, daily protein supply in, 63t
Electric pressure cooker, 121
Endotoxins, 60t
Environmental issues. See also Climate change/crisis; Greenhouse gas emissions
   animal agriculture's harm and, 49–50
   land use and, 43–44
   water consumption and, 45–48
   water pollution and, 48–49
   water quality and, 48–49
EPIC-Oxford Study (UK), 17t
Equal (sweetener), 20
Esophageal sphincter, 9
Essential fatty acids, 7, 59t
Ethanol production, corn and, 48
Exercise, 99–100, 104

F

Fajitas, Rainbow Veggie, 161–163
Falafel, 23, 85
   calories, protein, and the percentage of calories from protein, carbohydrates, and fat in, 32t
   Power Greens Salad, 138
Farmed fish. See Fish (farmed)
Farm subsidies, 43. See Subsidies, agricultural
Farro, 112, 122t
Fat(s)
   about, 7
   in animal products, 31
   in different types of milk, 77t
   limiting intake of, 104
   longevity and avoiding excess, 99
   in milk, 31
   percent of calories from, in milk, 31
   percent of calories in typical servings of various foods, 32–39t
   in plant foods, 32
   type 2 diabetes and, 55
Fat, percent of calories from, in typical servings of various foods, 32–39t
Fatty acids, 7, 101
Feed grains, 3, 4
Feedlots, 44
Fiber
   digestibility and, 12
   health gut microbiome and, 90
   meat alternatives and, 29
   in plant versus animal protein, 59t
   recommendations for plant-based eaters and, 14, 70
Field Roast Sausage, 32t, 33t
Figs, 37t
Finland, protein sources and type 2 diabetes in, 55

Fish (farmed)
  calories, protein, and the percentage of calories from protein, carbohydrates, and fat in, 39t
  greenhouse gas emissions and, 42f
  land use and, 45f
  water consumption and, 46, 47f
  water pollution and, 49f
Flaxseed oil, 101
Flaxseeds
  calories, protein, and the percentage of calories from protein, carbohydrates, and fat in, 33t
  Carrot Spice Cookies, 137
  Double-Chocolate Surprise Cookies, 135
  omega-3 fatty acids in, 101, 112
  protein, leucine, and lysine in, 24t
Flexitarian, 5
Food and Agriculture Organization (FAO), 4
  The Food Climate Research Network-Plates, Pyramids, Planet, 66–67
Food choices
  climate crisis and, 41–42
  tips for adding protein with your, 105–107
  using the Plant-Based Plate, 104
  water scarcity and, 45, 46
Food guides, 2
Food preparation
  added oil and, 115–116
  added salt and, 116–117
  added sugar and, 114–115
  cooking beans, 118–119
  cooking class for, 111
  cooking grains, 120–121
  digestibility and, 13–14
  electric pressure cooker for, 121
  essential kitchen equipment for, 110–111
  kitchen shortcuts for, 118–119

  plant-based pantry for, 111–114
  sourcing ingredients for, 111
  tips for using recipes, 117–118
Food security, 43–44
Forks Over Knives (documentary), 86
Formula, for babies. *See* Infant formula
Fortified milks, 76, 77t, 124
Fracking, 46
France
  cancer and protein sources in, 58
  daily protein supply in, 63t
  studies on protein intake in, 16, 17t
French Canadian Pea Soup, 105, 152
Fresh water, 46
Fruit(s). *See also* specific fruits
  calories, protein, and the percentage of calories from protein, carbohydrates, and fat in, 37–38t
  farm subsidies for, 3
  in the plant-based plate, 103t
  Powered-Up Overnight Oats, 125
  shifting subsidies to, 4
  for your pantry, 113
Full of Beans Salad, 105, 141

G

Gado Gado, 106, 169–170
Gado Gado Sauce, 151
The Game Changers (documentary), 79
Garbanzo beans. *See* Chickpeas (garbanzo)
Garlic cloves, 36t
Gelatin, 11, 19
Gender, plant-based diets and, 4, 5
Genetically modified (GMO) soy, 47, 48

Germany
  daily protein supply in, 63
  dietary guidelines of, 66
Ghana, daily protein supply in, 63t
Ginger, Lime, and Miso Dressing, 150, 164
Glutamate, 21
Glutamine, 20
Glycine, 20
Glycogen, 90
GMO-free soybeans, 47, 48
Golden Scrambled Tofu, 98, 106, 129
Gorilla Granola, 98, 106, 127–128
Government subsidies, 3–4
Grains. *See also* Whole grains
  calories, protein, and the percentage of calories from protein, carbohydrates, and fat in, 37–38t
  in plant-based plate, 103t
  presoaking, 118
  providing significant amounts of protein, leucine, and lysine, 24–25t
  tips for using higher-protein, 107
Granola. *See* Gorilla Granola
Grapefruit, 37t
Grapes, 37t
Grass-finished cattle, 44
Grasslands, 43–44
Great Northern beans, 32t, 112, 117
Green beans, in Gado Gado, 169–170
Greenhouse gas emissions
  from animal agriculture, 41
  disadvantaged countries impacted by, 42–43
  farm subsidies, 3
  food choices and, 41–42, 42f
  grass-finished cattle and, 44
  meat alternatives and, 28, 29

Green Power Smoothie, 98, 106, 124
Guatemala, daily protein supply in, 63t
Guava, 37t
Gut microbiome, 59t, 90

H

Hamilton, Lewis, 5
Harvard study, 95, 99
Hazelnuts. *See also* Nuts
  amino acids and, 23
  calories, protein, and the percentage of calories from protein, carbohydrates, and fat in, 37–38t
  protein, leucine, and lysine in, 24t
Health. *See also* Chronic disease(s)
  bone, 96
  long-term consequences of plant-based diet for children and, 81–82
  most protective sources of plant protein for your, 60–61
  plant protein advantage for, 58–59, 59–60t
  salt intake and, 116
  studies on protein sources and mortality, 51–53
Health Canada, 67
Heartburn, 9
Heart health
  plant-based diets and, 4–5
  protein overconsumption and, 16
  studies on protein sources and, 53–54
Hearty Vegetable Dahl, 166
Heatwaves, 45
Heme iron, 57, 60t
Hemoglobin, 7, 9
Hemp hearts, 34t
Hemp milk, 38t

Hemp seeds, 23, 61, 106
  calories, protein, and the percentage of calories from protein, carbohydrates, and fat in, 34t
  Carrot Spice Cookies, 137
  Double-Chocolate Surprise Cookies, 135
  Gorilla Granola, 127–128
  in Green Power Smoothie, 124
  Kale Salad with Orange-Ginger Dressing, 143
  Lemon-Tahini Protein-Plus Dressing, 148
  for omega-3 fatty acids, 101, 112
  Powered-Up Overnight Oats, 125
  protein, leucine, and lysine in, 24t
  Vanilla Chia Pudding, 134
Herbs and spices, in your pantry, 114
Herpes simplex virus, 21–22
Histidine, 19, 92
Hodgkin, Dorothy, 8
Honeydew melon, 37t
Hong Kong, daily protein supply in, 63t, 64
Hormel, 5
Hot dog, vegan, 32t, 33t
Hummus, 61, 83, 105
Hummus and Lime Dressing, 149
Hydration, 104
Hydrogen, 7, 8, 22f
Hypothyroidism, 27

I

IGF-1 (hormone), 96
Impossible Burgers, 29, 30
  calories, protein, and the percentage of calories from protein, carbohydrates, and fat in, 34t
  leghemoglobin in, 60t
Incomplete protein, 10–11
India, daily protein supply in, 63t

Infant formula, 73, 74, 76–77
Infants
  histidine and, 19
  protein needs, 73–74
  soy formula for, 76–77
Inflammation
  benefit of plant-protein foods for, 90
  exercise and, 99
Insulin, 8, 8f
Intergovernmental Panel on Climate Change (IPCC), 66
International reports, encouraging shift to plant-based diets, 65–67
International Society of Sport Nutrition, 25, 87, 88, 88t, 89, 94
International trade, farm subsidies and, 3
Iodine/iodine deficiency, 27, 104, 116
Iran
  cancer and protein sources in, 56
  mortality and protein sources in, 52
Iraq, daily protein supply in, 63t
Iron, 7, 76, 77t
Irving, Kyrie, 5
Isoflavones, 26–27, 56
Isoleucine, 9, 19, 22, 22f, 88–89, 93
Italy, daily protein supply in, 63t

J

Jamaica, daily protein supply in, 63t
Japan
  cancer and protein sources in, 57
  daily protein supply in, 63t
  mortality and plant *versus* animal protein diets in, 52
  soy consumed in, 27
The Jungle (Sinclair), 1

K

Kale. *See also* Leafy greens
    amino acids and, 23
    The Big Bowl, 164
    calories, protein, and the percentage of calories from protein, carbohydrates, and fat in, 36t
    Curry in a Hurry, 154
    Green Power Smoothie, 124
    Hearty Vegetable Dahl, 166
    Kale Salad with Orange-Ginger Dressing, 143
    Power Greens Salad, 138
    Rainbow Veggie Fajitas, 161–163
Kale Salad with Orange-Ginger Dressing, 106, 109t, 143
Kamut/Kamut berries. *See also* Whole grains
    calories, protein, and the percentage of calories from protein, carbohydrates, and fat in, 34t
    cooking times, 122t
    protein from, 107
    protein, leucine, and lysine in, 25t
Kelp, 36t, 104, 147
Kenya, daily protein supply in, 63t
Kidney beans. *See also* Beans
    calories, protein, and the percentage of calories from protein, carbohydrates, and fat in, 32t
    Easy-Peasy Chili, 156
    protein, leucine, and lysine in, 24t
Kidney disease, 92–93, 99
Kidneys, protein overconsumption and, 16, 96
Kiwifruit, 38t

L

Lactation
    benefits of plant-based diet during, 72
    protein needs and, 13, 70t

protein powders used during, 72
Lacto-ovo vegetarian diet, 17t, 74–75
Lamb
    greenhouse gas emissions and, 42f
    land use and, 44, 45f
    water consumption and, 47f
    water pollution and, 49f
Land use, 43–45
LDL cholesterol, 27, 55
Leafy greens. *See also* specific leafy greens
    The Big Bowl, 164
    Black Bean Stew, 159
    Curry in a Hurry, 154
    Gado Gado, 169–170
    Golden Scrambled Tofu and Veggies, 129
    Hearty Vegetable Dahl, 166
    in your pantry, 113
Leeks, 36t
Legume-based pastas, 61, 83, 105, 112, 144
Legumes. *See also* Beans; Chickpeas (garbanzo); Lentils; Peanuts
    benefits of, 100
    calories, protein, and the percentage of calories from protein, carbohydrates, and fat in, 32–33t
    cooking, 119–120
    digestibility and, 13–14
    eating three or more daily servings of, 105
    food preparation and digestibility of, 13–14
    getting children/teens to like, 84–85
    greenhouse gas emissions and, 42
    health benefits of, 61
    leucine from, 23

in the plant-based plate, 103t
    providing significant amounts of protein, leucine, and lysine, 24–25t
    raw, digestibility and, 13–14
    tips on using for meals and snacks, 105
    for toddler diet, 75
    water consumption and, 46
Lemon-Tahini Protein-Plus Dressing, 106, 109t
    for Power Greens Salad, 138
    recipe, 148
Lentils, 23, 24t
    calories, protein, and the percentage of calories from protein, carbohydrates, and fat in, 32t
    cooking, 119–120
    Curry in a Hurry, 154
    essential amino acids in, 19
    Hearty Vegetable Dahl, 166
    Lentil Tabbouleh, 142
    Power Greens Salad, 138
Lentil sprouts, 32t
Lentil Tabouleh, 142
Lettuce/mixed greens
    calories, protein, and the percentage of calories from protein, carbohydrates, and fat in, 36t
    Power Greens Salad, 138
Leucine, 9, 22
    in amino acid supplement, 93
    foods providing, 23, 24–25t
    function of, 19–20, 88–89
    muscle mass and, 97
    for plant-based athletes, 88–89
    recommended intake for seniors with special health conditions, 98–99
    for seniors, 97, 98
    structure of, 22f
Leucine supplements, 25, 26, 93
Lima beans, 24t, 32t

Liver
  amino acids and, 9
  protein overconsumption and, 16
Lobbyists, milk industry, 4
L-tryptophan supplement, 21
Lunch
  adding protein to, for muscle
    building, 83
  examples of simple protein
    boosts for, 91t
  menu ideas, 108t
  for seniors, 98
Lysine, 19, 20
  plant foods providing, 23, 24–25t
  supplemental, 21–22
  in toddler diet, 75

M

Macronutrients, 1, 7. See also Carbohydrates; Fat(s); Protein(s)
Males
  soy and feminization of, 76–77
  soy and prostate cancer of, 27
  soy intake and, 27
Malnutrition, 1
Mango
  calories, protein, and the percent-
    age of calories from protein,
    carbohydrates, and fat in, 38t
  Green Power Smoothie, 124
Maple Leaf, 5
Maple syrup
  calories, protein, and the percent-
    age of calories from protein,
    carbohydrates, and fat in, 38t
  Full of Beans Salad, 141
  Gorilla Granola, 127–128
  replacing sugar with, 115
  for your pantry, 114
Margarine, 38t
Meat alternatives
  about, 28, 30

comparing meat to advantages
  of, 29
downsides to, 29
as a healthy choice, 28–29
meat versus, 29
Meatballs (veggie), 23
Meat industry, farm subsidies and,
  2, 3–4
Meat Inspection Act, 1
Meat, meat alternatives versus, 29
Meatpacking industry, 1
Melina, Vesanto, 86
Menus, 107–109
Messenger RNA, 10
Methionine, 2, 19, 20
Mexico, daily protein supply in, 63t
Milk. See also Coconut milk;
    Cow's milk; Nondairy milk(s)
  breast, 72, 73–74
  fat in, 31
  greenhouse gas emissions and, 42f
  land use and, 45f
  nutritional comparison of vari-
    ous, 76, 77t
  for seniors, 98
  for toddlers, 76
  water consumption and, 46, 47f
  water pollution and, 49f
Millet
  calories, protein, and the percent-
    age of calories from protein,
    carbohydrates, and fat in, 34t
  cooking time, 122t
Miso
  Ginger, Lime, and Miso Dress-
    ing, 150
  Kale Salad with Orange-Ginger
    Dressing, 143
Miso-Mustard Tempeh, 130
Monocultures, 47, 48
Monosodium glutamate (MSG),
  21
Mung beans

calories, protein, and the percentage of calories from protein,
  carbohydrates, and fat in, 33t
Hearty Vegetable Dahl, 166
Mung bean sprouts
  calories, protein, and the percent-
    age of calories from protein,
    carbohydrates, and fat in, 33t
  Gado Gado, 169–170
Muscle building
  branched-chain amino acid snacks
    and meals for, 23
  branched-chain amino acid
    supplements and, 25
  for children and adolescents on
    plant-based diet, 82–83
  exercise and, 99–100
  plant protein as good as animal
    protein for, 26, 89
Muscle wasting, 15, 97. See also
    Sarcopenia (muscle wasting)
Mushrooms
  calories, protein, and the percent-
    age of calories from protein,
    carbohydrates, and fat in, 36t
  Creamy Mushroom-Broccoli
    Sauce, 167
  Golden Scrambled Tofu and
    Veggies, 129
  Rainbow Veggie Fajitas, 161–163
Mustard greens, 36t
Mutton
  greenhouse gas emissions and,
    42f
  land use and, 44, 45f
  water consumption and, 47f
  water pollution and, 49f
Myoglobin, 9

N

National Health and Nutrition
    Examination Survey, 16

National Institutes of Health, 26, 92

Nation Rising, 3

Natural pastures, 43–45

Navy beans, 75, 117
  calories, protein, and the percentage of calories from protein, carbohydrates, and fat in, 33*t*
  protein, leucine, and lysine in, 24*t*
  Stove-Top Baked Beans, 160

Nepal, daily protein supply in, 63*t*

Nestlé, 5

Netherlands, protein sources and type 2 diabetes in, 55

Neu5Gc, 60*t*

New Deal, 3

New Zealand, agricultural subsidies repealed in, 4

Nitrogen
  insulin molecule, 8
  protein overconsumption and, 16
  in proteins, 7

Nondairy beverages, 38*t*

Nondairy milk(s). *See also* specific nondairy milks
  calories, protein, and the percentage of calories from protein, carbohydrates, and fat in, 38*t*
  for children and teens, 82, 83
  Creamy Vanilla Chia Pudding, 134
  Green Power Smoothie, 124
  increase in sales of, 4
  Powered-Up Overnight Oats, 125
  tips for adding to meals, 105
  for toddlers, 76
  Vanilla Chia Pudding, 134

Nondairy products, in your pantry, 113

Nonessential amino acids, 11, 21, 92

Non-GMO soy, 47, 48

North American Adventist Health Study. *See* Adventist Health Study

North American Adventist Health Study-2 (AHS-2), 16, 17*t*

Nursing homes, 100

Nut butters. *See also* Peanut butter
  Carrot Spice Cookies, 137
  Double-Chocolate Surprise Cookies, 135
  Ginger, Lime, and Miso Dressing, 150
  as good source of protein, 61
  Gorilla Granola, 127–128
  making a part of your daily diet, 106–107
  sandwich snack using, 23
  thinning out, 137

NutraSweet, 20

Nutrinet-Santé Study (France), 17*t*

Nutritional yeast flakes, 117
  Creamy Mushroom-Broccoli Sauce, 167
  Golden Scrambled Tofu and Veggies, 129
  Lemon-Tahini Protein-Plus Dressing, 148
  Tangy Chickpea Smash, 147
  for Tofu Fingers, 133

Nuts. *See also* specific nuts
  calories, protein, and the percentage of calories from protein, carbohydrates, and fat in, 33–34*t*
  essential amino acids in, 19
  farm subsidies for, 3
  fresh water consumption and, 46, 47*f*
  greenhouse gas emissions and, 42*f*
  health benefits of, 61
  land use and, 45*f*
  leucine from, 23

making a part of your daily diet, 106–107
  in plant-based plate, 103*t*
  Powered-Up Overnight Oats, 125
  as source of fat, 104
  used instead of oils in dressings, 116
  water consumption and, 46, 47*f*
  water pollution and, 49*f*
  in your pantry, 112–113

O

Oat groats, 34*t*

Oat milk
  calories, protein, and the percentage of calories from protein, carbohydrates, and fat in, 38*t*
  compared with other milks, 77*t*

Oats and oatmeal
  calories, protein, and the percentage of calories from protein, carbohydrates, and fat in, 35*t*
  cooking times, 122*t*
  protein, leucine, and lysine in, 25*t*

Oats, rolled, 23
  calories, protein, and the percentage of calories from protein, carbohydrates, and fat in, 34*t*
  Carrot Spice Cookies, 137
  Gorilla Granola, 127–128
  Powered-Up Overnight Oats, 125

Oils
  calories, protein, and the percentage of calories from protein, carbohydrates, and fat in, 38*t*
  limiting intake of, 104
  tips for minimizing use of added, 115–116
  for your pantry, 114

Okinawan Japanese, 27

Okra, 36*t*

Oligosaccharides, 13, 119
Omega-3 fatty acids, 7
  sources of, 101, 103t, 112
Omega-6 fatty acids, 7
Omnivores, 28, 72, 92
Omnivorous diet
  getting too much protein with, 94
  protein intake in toddlers on a,
    74–75
  protein intakes of plant-based
    youth compared with youth
    on a, 80–81
Onions n, 36t
Orange-Ginger Dressing, 143
Orange juice
  calories, protein, and the percent-
    age of calories from protein,
    carbohydrates, and fat in, 38t
  Orange-Ginger Dressing, 143
Oranges
  calories, protein, and the percent-
    age of calories from protein,
    carbohydrates, and fat in, 38t
  Gorilla Granola, 127–128
Overnight Oat, 125
Oxidative stress, 59t, 60t, 90
Oxygen, 7, 8

P

Pantry, plant-based, 111–114
Papaya, 38t
Parsnips, 36t
Pasta
  calories, protein, and the percent-
    age of calories from protein,
    carbohydrates, and fat in, 35t
  legume-based, 61, 83, 105, 112,
    144
  lentil, 33t
  Peanut-Edamame Noodle Salad,
    144
  whole wheat, 25t, 35t

PDCAAS (Protein Digestibility
    Corrected Amino Acid Score),
    11–12
Peaches, 38t
Pea milk, 38t, 77t, 113
Peanut butter
  calories, protein, and the percent-
    age of calories from protein,
    carbohydrates, and fat in, 33t
  for children/teens, 82, 83
  Double-Chocolate Surprise
    Cookies, 135
  Gado Gado Sauce, 151
  as good source of protein,
    106–107
  Peanut-Edamame Noodle Salad,
    144
  as protein booster in Green
    Power Smoothie, 124
  snack made with, 23
  on toast for breakfast, 98
Peanut-Edamame Noodle Salad, 144
Peanuts, 23. *See also* Peanut butter
  calories, protein, and the percent-
    age of calories from protein,
    carbohydrates, and fat in, 33t
  essential amino acids in, 19
  greenhouse gas emissions and, 42f
  land use and, 45f
  as part of your daily diet, 106
  Peanut-Edamame Noodle Salad,
    144
  protein, leucine, and lysine in, 24t
  snack made from, 83
  water consumption and, 46, 47f
  water pollution and, 49f
Pea pods, 36t
Pears, 38t
Peas
  calories, protein, and the percent-
    age of calories from protein,
    carbohydrates, and fat in, 33t,
    36t

cooking, 119–120
Creamy Mushroom-Broccoli
  Sauce, 167
essential amino acids in, 19
greenhouse gas emissions and,
  42f
land use and, 45f
as protein booster in Green
  Power Smoothie, 124
water consumption and, 47f
water pollution and, 49f
Pea sprouts, 33t
Pecans. *See also* Nuts
  calories, protein, and the per-
    centage of calories from pro-
    tein, carbohydrates, and fat
    in, 34t
  Carrot Spice Cookies, 137
  protein, leucine, and lysine in,
    24t
Peppers (bell)
  The Big Bowl, 164
  calories, protein, and the percent-
    age of calories from protein,
    carbohydrates, and fat in, 36t
  Creamy Mushroom-Broccoli
    Sauce, 167
  Curry in a Hurry, 154
  Easy-Peasy Chili, 156–158
  Full of Beans Salad, 141
  Gado Gado, 169–170
  Golden Scrambled Tofu and
    Veggies, 129
  Hearty Vegetable Dahl, 166
  Kale Salad with Orange-Ginger
    Dressing, 143
  Peanut-Edamame Noodle Salad,
    144
  Rainbow Veggie Fajitas, 161–163
Pepsin, 9
Peptides, 9
Perdue, 5
Phenylalanine, 19, 20

Philippines, daily protein supply in, 63t
Physical activity, 99–100, 104
Phytochemicals, 59t
Pineapple
    calories, protein, and the percentage of calories from protein, carbohydrates, and fat in, 38t
    in Green Power Smoothie, 124
Pine nuts, 23
Pinto beans. *See also* Beans
    calories, protein, and the percentage of calories from protein, carbohydrates, and fat in, 38t
    Easy Peasy Chili, 156
    protein, leucine, and lysine in, 24t
Pistachio nuts, 61
    calories, protein, and the percentage of calories from protein, carbohydrates, and fat in, 38t
    protein, leucine, and lysine in, 24t
Plant-based athletes. *See* Athletes
Plant-based diet
    advantages over animal protein, 90
    branched-chain amino acids in a, 23, 25
    breastfeeding and, 73–74
    challenges of children and adolescents on, 82–85
    for children and teens, 79
    "conditionally essential" amino acids and, 20
    gender and, 4
    heart health and, 4–5
    international reports/organizations encouraging a, 64–68
    during pregnancy, 69–70, 72
    protein digestibility and, 12–13
    protein intake on, 51
Plant-based foods. *See also* specific foods
    agricultural subsidies and, 3, 4

amino acids provided by, 10, 21
calcium losses and, 96
carbohydrates from, 7
essential amino acids in, 19
high-leucine, 23
"incomplete protein" concept and, 10–11
meat alternatives, 28–30
providing significant amounts of protein, leucine, and lysine, 24–25t
water consumption and, 47–48
in your pantry, 111–114
Plant-based milk. *See* Nondairy milk(s)
Plant-Based Plate, 11, 75, 101–103, 102f, 103t
Plant enzymes, 59t
Plant protein
    advantages of athletes swapping animal protein for, 90
    digestibility of, 12–13
    global supply, 63t, 64
    health impact of animal protein *versus*, 51–53, 58–59, 59–60t
    most protective sources of, 60–61
    muscle building and, 26, 89
Plant sterols, 59t
Plums, 38t
Poppy seeds, 34t
Pork
    greenhouse gas emissions and, 42f
    land use and, 45f
    water consumption and, 46
    water pollution and, 49f
Portugal, daily protein supply in, 63t
Potatoes
    amino acids and, 23
    calories, protein, and the percentage of calories from protein, carbohydrates, and fat in, 36t

Veggie Sausage and Sauerkraut Soup, 153
Potato protein, in protein powders, 93
Poultry
    greenhouse gas emissions and, 42, 42f
    land use and, 45f
    water consumption and, 46, 47f
Powered-Up Overnight Oats, 125
Power Greens Salad, 109t, 138
Prawns (farmed)
    greenhouse gas emissions and, 42f
    land use and, 45f
    water consumption and, 46, 47f
    water pollution and, 49f
Prebiotics, 59t
Pregnancy
    benefits of plant-based diet during, 72
    menu ideas for, 109t
    protein needs, 13, 69–72
    protein powders used during, 72
    recommended protein intake during, 108
Probiotics, 59t
Proline, 21
Protein(s). *See also* Animal protein; Plant protein
    about, 7
    absorption of, 12
    activities accomplished by various, 6–7
    athletes getting too much, 94
    calculating percent of calories coming from, 15
    calculating your recommended intake of, 14
    complementation for toddlers, 75
    concept of complete and incomplete, 10–11
    in different types of milk, 77t

digestibility of, 11–13
focus on malnutrition from, 2
getting too much, 16–17
insulin molecule, 8–9
in legumes and products, 32–33t
life cycle of a, 9–10
molecular weight of, 8
percent of calories in typical servings of various foods, 32–39t
quiz about, 6, 18
signs of deficiency in, 15
studies on intake of, 16, 17t
synthesis, 10
word origin, 6
Protein intake
bone health and high, 96
health impact of excessive, 51
for infants, 73–74
muscle wasting and, 97
of plant-based toddlers versus omnivorous toddlers, 74–75
of plant-based youth versus omnivorous youth, 80–81
during pregnancy, 69–72
recommended for athletes, 87–88, 88t, 108t
recommended for seniors, 97, 98–99, 108
for seniors, 97
for seniors with special health conditions, 98–99
studies on, 16, 17t
timing of, for athletes, 89
for toddlers, 78
Protein needs
for athletes, 13, 87–88, 88t
during childhood and adolescence, 13, 80–81, 81t
for infants, 73–74
during pregnancy, 13, 69–72, 71t
for seniors, 13
for toddlers, 13, 73, 74

as we age, 96
Protein powders, 107
for plant-based athletes, 93–94
as protein booster in Green Power Smoothie, 124
used during pregnancy and lactation, 72
Protein quality, 2
Protein-rich foods, 23. See also Plant protein; specific foods
advantages of plant-based versus animal products, 90
animal products and, 31, 99
to build into meals or snacks, 23
to build muscle or lean body mass, 23
Canadian dietary guidelines on, 67
featured in meals and snacks, 107
longevity by replacing animal with plant-based, 99
meals and snacks for athletes, 89, 91, 91t
meals and snacks for seniors, 97–98
in the plant-based plate, 103t
for pregnancy, 60–61
quiz on, 31, 39
Protein supplements
for athletes, 93
during pregnancy, 72
Protein supply, statistics on global, 62, 63t, 64
Protein synthesis, 10
branched-chain amino acids and, 88–89
branched-chain amino acid supplements and, 25
timing of protein intake and, 89
Prunes, 38t
Puberty, 82
Pumpkin Pie Spice

in Carrot Spice Cookies, 137
recipe, 137
Pumpkin seeds, 23, 61, 106
calories, protein, and the percentage of calories from protein, carbohydrates, and fat inn, 34t
Gorilla Granola, 127–128
Kale Salad with Orange-Ginger Dressing, 143
protein, leucine, and lysine in, 24t
Pure Food and Drug Act, 1

Q
Qatar, dietary guidelines in, 67
Quinoa, 122t. See also Whole grains
calories, protein, and the percentage of calories from protein, carbohydrates, and fat in, 35t
cooking time, 122t
essential amino acids in, 19
protein, leucine, and lysine in, 25t
Quinoa with peas, 23

R
Radishes, 36t
Rainbow Veggie Fajitas, 106, 161–163
Raisins
calories, protein, and the percentage of calories from protein, carbohydrates, and fat in, 38t
Carrot Spice Cookies, 137
Gorilla Granola, 127–128
Powered-Up Overnight Oats, 125
Raspberries, 38t
Raw cashews
Creamy Mushroom-Broccoli Sauce, 167
in your pantry, 112

Recommended dietary allowance (RDA)
  of calcium, 96
  for children aged 4-13 years old, 80
  for leucine, 23
  for lysine in toddlers, 75–76
  for plant-based eaters, 14
  of protein for children and adolescents, 13, 80–81, 81t
  of protein for infants, 74
  of protein for plant-based eaters, 14
  of protein for teens, 80
  of protein for toddlers, 13, 74
  protein needs during pregnancy, 13, 69, 70t, 71, 71t
  for vitamin D, 104
Research. See Studies
Rice. See also Brown rice; White rice; Wild rice
  cooking times, 122t
  greenhouse gas emissions and, 42f
  incomplete protein and, 11
  land use and, 45f
  lysine and, 20, 75–76
  protein from, 107
  water consumption and, 46, 47f
  water pollution and, 49f
  in your pantry, 112
Rice-based diets, 11, 20
Rice milk, 38t
Rice with beans, 23, 84
RNA molecules, 10
Rolled oats. See Oats, rolled
Roll, Rich, 5
Rutabaga, 36t
Rye
  greenhouse gas emissions and, 42f
  land use and, 45f
  water consumption and, 47f
  water pollution and, 49f
Rye berries, 122t

S
Sacred Cow (documentary), 47
Salad dressings. See Dressings
Salads
  Full of Beans Salad, 141
  Kale Salad with Orange-Ginger Dressing, 143
  Peanut-Edamame Noodle Salad, 144
  Power Greens Salad, 138
Salmon, 39t
Salt
  health issues with, 116
  tips for decreasing, 116–117
Samoa, daily protein supply in, 63t, 64
Sarcopenia (muscle wasting), 19–20, 97
  leucine and, 19–20
  protein needs and, 13
  recommended protein and leucine intake for, 98–99
Saturated fat
  in plant versus animal protein, 60t
  type 2 diabetes and, 55
Sauces
  Creamy Mushroom-Broccoli Sauce, 167
  Gado Gado Sauce, 151
Sauerkraut, in Veggie Sausage and Sauerkraut Soup, 153
Seal-eating populations, 11
Sea vegetables, 104
Seed butters, 61
  Double-Chocolate Surprise Cookies, 135
  Gorilla Granola, 127–128
Seeds

calories, protein, and the percentage of calories from protein, carbohydrates, and fat in, 33–34t
essential amino acids in, 19
health benefits of, 61
leucine from, 23
in plant-based plate, 103t
providing significant amounts of protein, leucine, and lysine, 24–25t
as source of fats, 104
tips on using for meals and snacks, 106
used instead of oils in dressings, 116
in your pantry, 112–113
Seitan, 61, 89
  calories, protein, and the percentage of calories from protein, carbohydrates, and fat in, 35t
  protein, leucine, and lysine in, 25t
Selenium, 20
Selenium-containing proteins, 7, 20
Seniors and aging
  bone health and, 96
  exercise and, 99–100
  menu ideas for, 109t
  muscle wasting and, 97
  protein deficiency and, 15
  protein needs, 13
  protein-rich meals and snacks for, 97–98
  recommended protein intake for, 97, 98–99, 108
Serine, 21
Serum albumin, 15
Serving sizes, 101
Sesame seeds
  The Big Bowl, 164
  calories, protein, and the percentage of calories from protein, carbohydrates, and fat in, 34t

Sesame tahini. *See also* Tahini
  calories, protein, and the percentage of calories from protein, carbohydrates, and fat in, 34t
  protein, leucine, and lysine in, 24t
Seventh-day Adventists, Loma Linda, California, 27
Smithfield, 5
Smoothie, Green Power, 98, 106, 124
Snacks
  adding protein to, 83
  before bedtime, for resistance training, 89
  examples of simple protein boosts for, 91t
  ideas for, 108t
  protein-rich, 23, 107
  for seniors, 98
Soaking legumes, 13, 118–119
Social justice issues, 42–43
Sodium consumption, 104
Sorghum, 122t
Soups
  French Canadian Pea Soup, 152
  Veggie Sausage and Sauerkraut Soup, 153
South Korea
  cancer and protein sources in, 57
  daily protein supply in, 63t
Soybean production, 47–48
Soybeans, 23
  calories, protein, and the percentage of calories from protein, carbohydrates, and fat in, 33t
  farm subsidies for, 3
Soy foods
  criticism of soybean production and, 47–48

effects of isoflavones in, 26–27
essential amino acids in, 19
during pregnancy, 72
rumors about, 27
safety of, 27–28
for toddlers, 76–77
Soy formula, 73, 76–77
Soy milk, 23, 27, 70, 72, 75, 113
  for babies and toddlers, 76–77
  calories, protein, and the percentage of calories from protein, carbohydrates, and fat in, 38t
  Creamy Mushroom-Broccoli Sauce, 167
  greenhouse gas emissions and, 42f
  in Green Power Smoothie, 124
  land use and, 45f
  nutrition in, 77t
  Powered-Up Overnight Oats, 125
  protein for seniors through, 98
  for toddlers, 76
  water consumption and, 47f
  water pollution and, 49f
Soy protein isolate, 12
Soy protein powder, 24t
Spaghetti (whole wheat), 23
Spain, daily protein supply in, 63t
Spelt/spelt berries
  calories, protein, and the percentage of calories from protein, carbohydrates, and fat in, 35t
  cooking times, 122t
  protein from, 107
  protein, leucine, and lysine in, 25t
Spinach. *See also* Leafy greens
  amino acids and, 23
  calories, protein, and the percentage of calories from protein, carbohydrates, and fat in, 35t
  Curry in a Hurry, 154

Hearty Vegetable Dahl, 166
Split peas, 24t, 61. *See also* Legumes
  French Canadian Pea Soup, 152
Squash, 36–37t
Stove-Top Baked Beans, 105, 160
Strawberries
  calories, protein, and the percentage of calories from protein, carbohydrates, and fat in, 35t
  in Green Power Smoothie, 124
Studies. *See also* Adventist Health Study
  on breast milk, 72
  on digestibility and absorption of protein, 11–12
  on increasing longevity, 95–96, 99
  on muscle building, 99
  on plant *versus* animal protein for bone health, 16
  on plant *versus* animal protein for muscle building, 26
  on protein intake of plant-based youth versus omnivorous youth, 80–81
  on protein intakes in the UK, France, and North America, 16, 17t
  on protein intakes of toddlers aged one to three, 74–75
  on protein sources and cancer, 56–58
  on protein sources and cardiovascular disease, 53–54
  on protein sources and mortality, 51–53
  on protein sources and type 2 diabetes, 55–56
Subsidies, agricultural, 2
  Canadian, 3–4
  environmental impact, 3, 4
  international trade and, 3

shifting from animal products to plant foods, 3, 4
social justice and, 43
Sugar
calories, protein, and the percentage of calories from protein, carbohydrates, and fat in, 38t
in flavored milks, 76
limiting intake of, 104
Sunflower seed butter
calories, protein, and the percentage of calories from protein, carbohydrates, and fat in, 38t
Ginger, Lime, and Miso Dressing, 150
Sunflower seeds
calories, protein, and the percentage of calories from protein, carbohydrates, and fat in, 38t
Kale Salad with Orange-Ginger Dressing, 143
protein, leucine, and lysine in, 24t
Sunflower sprouts, 124
Sunlight, exposure to, 104
Supplements
amino acid, 9, 21–22, 92–93
for athletes, 92–93
branched-chain amino acids, 9, 25–26, 93, 99
iodine, 104
leucine, 25, 26, 93
protein, during pregnancy, 72
vitamin D, 97, 102, 104
Sustainable Healthy Diets: Guiding Principles (WHO/FAO), 65–66
Sweden, dietary guidelines, 66
Sweetened milk, 76, 77t
Sweeteners
calories, protein, and the percentage of calories from protein, carbohydrates, and fat in, 38t

in your pantry, 114
Sweet potato
calories, protein, and the percentage of calories from protein, carbohydrates, and fat in, 37t
Gado Gado, 169–170
Swiss Food Pyramid, 67–68

T
Tahini. See also Sesame tahini
Gado Gado Sauce, 151
Lemon-Tahini Protein-Plus Dressing, 148
Orange-Ginger Dressing, 143
Tangy Chickpea Smash, 147
Tangy Chickpea Smash, 147
Tasty Tofu Fingers, 98, 106, 132–133, 138
Teens. See Children and teens
Teff, 122t
Tempeh, 23, 27, 61
calories, protein, and the percentage of calories from protein, carbohydrates, and fat in, 33t
Gado Gado, 169–170
Power Greens Salad, 138
suggestions for using, 105–106
Tempting Tempeh, 130, 138
Tempting Tempeh, 130, 138
Thailand, daily protein supply in, 63t, 64
Threonine, 19, 20
TMAO (trimethylamine-N-oxide), 29, 60t
Toddlers
protein needs, 13, 73, 74
serving sizes for, 101
Tofu, 23, 27
calories, protein, and the percentage of calories from protein, carbohydrates, and fat in, 33t

Golden Scrambled Tofu and Veggies, 129
greenhouse gas emissions and, 42, 42f
health benefits of, 61
land use and, 44, 45f
as protein booster in Green Power Smoothie, 124
protein digestibility and, 12
protein, leucine, and lysine in, 24t
Rainbow Veggie Fajitas, 161–163
soybean production and, 47–48
suggestions for using, 105–106
Tasty Tofu Fingers, 132–133
water consumption and, 46, 47f
water pollution and, 48–49, 49f
Tomatoes
calories, protein, and the percentage of calories from protein, carbohydrates, and fat in, 37t
Easy-Peasy Chili, 156–158
Hearty Vegetable Dahl, 166
Lentil Tabbouleh, 142
prepping, 119
Tortillas, 34t, 35t
Rainbow Veggie Fajitas, 161–163
Transfer RNA, 10
Tree nut butters. See Nut butters
Tree nuts, 3, 106–107. See also Nuts
True Ileal Digestibility, 11, 12
Trypsin, 9
Trypsin inhibitors, 12, 14
Tryptophan, 11, 19, 20
Turkey, daily protein supply in, 63t
Turnip greens, 37t
Turnips, 37t
Type 2 diabetes, 55–56
Tyrosine, 20, 21

Tyson, 5

U

United Kingdom, studies on protein intake in, 16, 17t
United Nations Environmental Programme, 41
United Nations, Food and Agriculture Organization (FAO), 4, 41, 43, 65–66
United States
    cancer and protein sources in, 57
    cardiovascular disease and plant versus animal protein in, 53, 54
    daily protein supply in, 63t
    farm subsidies in, 3, 43
    "grass finished" cattle in, 44
    protein sources and type 2 diabetes in, 56
    studies on mortality and plant versus animal protein diets in, 52–53
    studies on protein intake in, 16, 17t

V

Valine, 9, 19, 22, 22f, 88–89
Vanilla almond milk, 76
VeChi Diet Study (Germany), 74–75, 80
Vegan crumbles
    calories, protein, and the percentage of calories from protein, carbohydrates, and fat in, 33t
    Easy-Peasy Chili, 156–158
Vegetables. See also specific vegetables
    boosters in Green Power Smoothie, 124

calories, protein, and the percentage of calories from protein, carbohydrates, and fat in, 35–37t
    in Curry in a Hurry, 154
    farm subsidies for, 3
    in the plant-based plate, 103t
    in Power Greens Salad, 138
    prepping, 119
    protein in, 107
    shifting subsidies to, 4
    for your pantry, 113
Vegetarian Resource Group, 100
Veggie burgers, 5, 23, 106
Veggie meats, 23, 61
    during pregnancy, 72
    for seniors, 98
    suggestions for use of, 106, 107
    for toddlers, children, and teens, 74, 83, 84
    in your pantry, 112
Veggie Sausage and Sauerkraut Soup, 153
Vietnam, daily protein supply in, 63t, 64
Vitamin A, 77t
Vitamin B12, 20, 76, 77t, 81, 97, 102, 105
Vitamin D, 76
    bone health and, 96
    low intakes among vegan youth, 81
    in milk, 77t, 105
    muscle mass and, 97
    recommendations for, 102, 104
    soy milk and, 98
    supplements, 97, 102, 104
Vitamins and minerals
    elimination of deficiency diseases and, 2
    fat-soluble, 7, 32
    first identification of, 1

supplements for pregnancy, 72
vegan diet for children and, 81

W

Walnuts, 61, 112. See also Nuts
    calories, protein, and the percentage of calories from protein, carbohydrates, and fat in, 34t
    Carrot Spice Cookies, 137
    Double-Chocolate Surprise Cookies, 135
    omega-3 fatty acids from, 101
    protein, leucine, and lysine in, 24t
Water chestnuts, 34t
Water consumption, 45–48
Watercress greens, 37t
Watermelon, 38t
Water quality, 48–50
Weight-bearing exercise, bone health and, 96
Wheat. See also Seitan
    greenhouse gas emissions and, 42f
    land use and, 45f
    water consumption and, 47f
    water pollution and, 49f
Wheat berries, cooking time for, 122t
Wheat sprouts, 35t
Wheat tortilla, 35t
White beans, 23, 33t, 117
White rice
    calories, protein, and the percentage of calories from protein, carbohydrates, and fat in, 35t
    protein, leucine, and lysine in, 25t
Whole grains. See also specific whole grains
    The Big Bowl, 164
    cooking, 120–121, 122t
    essential amino acids from, 19, 25

in the Plant-Based Plate, 103*t*, 104
in your pantry, 112
Whole wheat bread, 23, 25*t*, 34*t*
Whole wheat pasta/spaghetti, 25*t*,
    35*t*
Wild rice, 112
    calories, protein, and the percent-
        age of calories from protein,
        carbohydrates, and fat in, 35*t*

cooking time, 122*t*
essential amino acids in, 19
World Health Organization, 48,
    56, 65–66, 115
Worldwatch Institute, 41

Y

Yam, 37*t*

Z

Zambia, daily protein supply in,
    63*t*, 64
Zinc, 7, 20, 112
Zucchini
    calories, protein, and the percent-
        age of calories from protein,
        carbohydrates, and fat in, 37*t*
    Rainbow Veggie Fajitas, 161–163

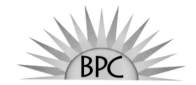

BPC

books that educate, inspire, and empower

To find your favorite books on plant-based cooking and nutrition,
raw-foods cuisine, and healthy living, visit
BookPubCo.com.

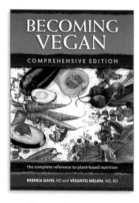

Becoming Vegan
Comprehensive Edition
Brenda Davis, RD, and Vesanto Melina, MS, RD
978-1-57067-297-2 • $34.95

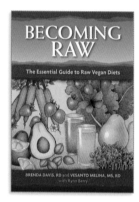

Becoming Raw
The Essential Guide to Raw Vegan Diets
Brenda Davis, RD, and Vesanto Melina, MS, RD
978-1-57067-238-5 • $24.95

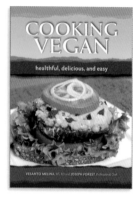

Cooking Vegan
Healthful, Delicious, Easy
Vesanto Melina, MS, RD, and Joseph Forest
978-1-57067-267-5 • $19.95

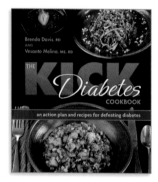

The Kick Diabetes Cookbook
An Action Plan and Recipes
for Defeating Diabetes
Brenda Davis, RD, and Vesanto Melina, MS, RD
978-1-57067-359-7 • $19.95

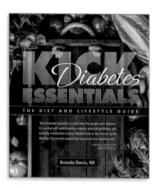

Kick Diabetes Essentials
The Diet and Lifestyle Guide
Brenda Davis, RD
978-1-57067-376-4 • $27.95

Purchase these titles from your favorite book source or buy them directly from
BPC • PO Box 99 • Summertown, TN 38483 • 1-888-260-8458
Free shipping and handling on all orders